P9-BIV-406

**MacGregor's Book
Nook Discard**
202 North Main Street
Yreka, CA 96097
(530) 841-2664

The
Surgical
Arena

The Surgical Arena

A NOVEL

PETER GRANT, M.D.

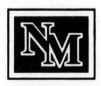

NEWMARK PUBLISHING COMPANY

Copyright © 1993 by Peter Grant, M.D.

All rights reserved including the right of reproduction
in whole or in part in any form.
Written permission must be obtained from the publisher.

Published in 1994 by
Newmark Publishing Company
South Windsor, Connecticut 06074
(203) 282-7265

Designed by Irving Perkins Associates, Inc.
Typeset by Pagesetters Incorporated
Printed and Bound by The Book Press
Manufactured in the United States of America

10 9 8 7 6 5 4 3 2 1

Library of Congress Cataloging-in-Publication Data

Grant, Peter, M.D.
The Surgical Arena
ISBN 0-938539-11-6   93-084589

"I *will not use the knife on sufferers from stone, but I will give place to such as are craftsmen therein.*"

THE OATH OF HIPPOCRATES
485 B.C.

"Ye *shall not cause any man injury by hastening to cut through flesh and blood with an iron instrument or by branding.*"

THE OATH OF ASAPH
AND COCHANAN
Sixth Century A.D.

"A *surgeon must be intelligent, compassionate and mentally in control at all times, for his hands can preserve life or destroy it.*"

ANONYMOUS
1993 A.D.

Author's Note

This is a work of fiction. The names, characters, and incidents are fictitious and entirely imaginary. Any resemblance to actual persons living or dead is strictly coincidental.

The
Surgical
Arena

Prologue

1984

JOYCE, CLAUDETTE, LILLIAN, AND JANE sat on the edge of the operating room stretchers, relaxing before the day's schedule began. Each head nurse had an operating room to run. It was 7:30 A.M. In their operating rooms they had prepared tables with sterile instruments designated for each case, packaged and covered with sterile drapes. While the four nurses sat on the stretchers chatting, the anesthesiologists were in the rooms checking the anesthesia equipment, drawing medications into sterile syringes. They were reviewing the charts of the patients, checking the blood work, EKGs, chest x-rays, and the medical histories and physicals.

"Looks like our population is aging," said Joe Morrone, one of the resident anesthesiologists.

"Yup," remarked the senior anesthesiologist. "Everyone gets a little bit older as the day passes by."

"That's a profound statement," replied Joe. "The only trouble is, the surgeons are operating on patients who are much older and we have to keep them alive during the operations. Someday there'll be an age limit for surgery."

"Forget it," said Charlie. "There are more old geezers than there are of us. And they have the AARP on their side."

Joe hollered out to Joyce, who was still sitting on the stretcher, "Hey, Joyce, where's Mr. Clean? Have you seen him yet?"

"No," she said. "But he'll be here on time. You know that."

Claudette spoke up. "How'd your surgeon get that nickname?"

"He hates the sight of blood," said Joyce. "He rarely has to use any blood on his cases, unlike Digger or the Grim Reaper."

"Digger? I'm almost afraid to ask which one of the surgeons is Digger."

"You know who I mean. He's the one who's always operating on fat patients."

"Thanks," said Claudette.

"He's got the biggest paws I've ever seen," said Joyce. "He looks like a dog digging for a bone."

"He's not as bad as Dr. Rush, the Grim Reaper," said Lillian. "I had him in my room two weeks ago and everything went wrong. He's bad news. He's impossible! He should have been a dermatologist or a psychiatrist or, better still, an undertaker. I don't let him work in my room anymore."

"How do you clear that with the supervisor?" asked Claudette.

"I have a tantrum," she said. "I scream and kick my feet and knock things over when they try to book him in my room. Two weeks ago, we had a routine thyroid case to do on an attractive twenty-eight-year-old female. He said it was routine. At least that's what *he* called it. I was going to speak up and say that none of his cases were routine, but I thought better of it. He started questioning his intern and resident in the scrub room, acting like a professor. 'Why do we operate on young women with single nodules in the thyroid?' he asked. 'Because they have a high incidence of cancer,' said the intern. 'That's right,' said Rush. 'What's the percentage?' 'It depends on whom you read,' replied the intern. 'Hmmm, clever answer,' said Dr. Rush. 'Well, make an estimate then.' 'I'd say eight percent,' replied the intern. 'Not bad,' said Rush. 'I'll accept that.' After scrubbing for ten minutes, he came into my operating room. The patient's neck was prepped and draped and a midline collar incision was made. It wasn't long before all hell broke loose."

The nurses leaned forward and listened intently.

"What happened?" asked Jane.

"Well, Rush was in a teaching mood and he wasn't watching what he was doing. He cut the strap muscles in the neck and then had the resident retract the thyroid lobe so he could locate the nerve that they try to avoid."

"You mean the recurrent laryngeal?" asked Joyce. "If you cut it, the patient can develop an airway obstruction and get hoarse because only one vocal chord moves. It can close down the windpipe."

"That's right, smarty," said Claudette. "And you can call in the lawyers when that happens. It's good for a malpractice case and it's big bucks."

"So, did he cut the nerve?" asked Joyce.

"No, better than that," said Lillian.

"Well, let's hear it. You're keeping us in suspense."

"He was meticulously dissecting, looking for the nerve, and he decided to tie off the middle thyroid vein that connects to the thyroid lobe. The resident was holding the clamp and he had a tie around it, but Rush pulled too hard in tying the silk suture and he tore a hole in the internal jugular vein."

"Oh, God," said Joyce.

"He put pressure on the hole in the vein with his finger and started screaming about the possibility of an air embolis. A lot of blood started filling the wound and he asked for a bigger tip for the metal sucker to suck out the blood. The anesthesiologist told me to call the blood bank for blood and then the shit really hit the fan."

"What happened?" asked Claudette.

"The patient wasn't typed and cross-matched for blood."

"Who the hell goofed?"

"It turned out the intern forgot to order the blood," said Lillian.

"Scratch one intern," said Joyce. "You always order extra blood for the Grim Reaper."

"That's right," said Lillian. "But wait, it gets better. Dr. Rush started screaming at the intern to pull the retractors harder so he could see where the hole was in the vein. 'Pull that retractor harder!' he yelled. Finally, after three pints of blood, he found the hole in the vein and sewed it up. I think the patient went into shock a few times."

"What's next?" asked Claudette.

"Well, he hadn't located the nerve yet and by this time his own nerves were a little frazzled. His hands started to shake. Finally, the surgical resident got up enough nerve and asked if he should take over. Rush looked up at him with as much dignity as he could, and said, 'Would you?' The resident found the nerve and they were able to remove the thyroid lobe with the tumor in it."

"What did they find?"

"It was a benign follicular cellular adenoma," said Lillian. "Anyway, it wasn't a cancer."

"So what's wrong with that?" asked Claudette.

"You haven't heard the end of the story," said Lillian. "The calamity on Fifth Avenue is just beginning. When the wound was closed and the anesthesia was stopped the patient didn't wake up."

"What do you mean?"

"Just what I said. The patient didn't wake up!"

"You mean she *died*?"

"No. The anesthesiologist had trouble getting her to breathe and respond."

"What happened?"

"The patient couldn't speak or move one of her arms."

"I still don't get it," said Joyce.

"She had a stroke while she was under anesthesia."

"A stroke at twenty-eight?"

"Yep. That's right. But it's not what you think."

"This is getting to be a real whodunnit," said Joyce.

"When they got her into the recovery room, they called in a neurologist and a neurosurgeon. Ben White, the neurosurgeon, examined the patient thoroughly. He's that real sharp new guy. And he said, 'You'd better call in a vascular surgeon, immediately! I can't feel a pulse in her left carotid artery.' "

"I'm lost," said Joyce.

"What happened was that when Dr. Rush got into trouble and tore a hole in the internal jugular vein, he hollered at the intern to pull hard on the retractors, which he did while they were trying to sew up the hole. With all that tugging and pressure on the carotid artery with the metal retractors, the patient got a blood clot in the artery, causing a stroke."

"What a disaster," said Joyce. "The Reaper could screw up a boiled egg."

"The vascular surgeon reoperated and cleaned out the clot in the artery but the damage was already done, and this twenty-eight-year-old girl now has permanent brain damage."

"Now I understand why they call him the Grim Reaper," said Joyce.

"All these surgeons have been nicknamed by the surgical residents," said Claudette. "There's a Bow Wow, Scary Harry, Slow Motion, Big Balls, Chief Honshu, Cry Baby, Chop Sticks, Big Mac, Grim Reaper, Popeye, Stud, and Mickey Mouse."

"I'd love to hear the stories behind those names," said Joyce.

"Here comes Mr. Clean now," said Claudette. "He's still a good-looking hunk of meat, for a white man."

"I'm sure you wouldn't kick him out of bed if he crawled in with you. I don't think Clean would cross the color line," said Joyce.

"Shut your mouth. Twenty years ago, I'd have no trouble wrestling with him, black or white."

Joyce laughed as she said, "You'd better be quiet, he might hear you."

"He's your boss, not mine, honey."

"Yeah, and he's got seven hours booked today," said Joyce.

"What's he doing?" asked Jane.

"He's got a big head and neck cancer case, and also a breast cancer case."

"Well, I hope you get a coffee break," said Claudette.

"Morning, Joyce," said Dr. Kendall. "We've got an interesting schedule today."

"I noticed," said Joyce.

"There'll be some visiting surgeons in to watch the first case. It's a head and neck vascular tumor problem."

"Haven't we done that patient before?" asked Joyce.

"Yes," said Dr. Kendall. "Mr. Gordon flew in from St. Louis. He's a VP with that big aircraft company out there. He's got a recurrent carotid body tumor. It's a blood vessel and glandular tumor and it can be a bloody mess. Hopefully, it won't be," said Matt. "We had the tumor embolized."

"What do you mean?" asked Joyce.

"Two days ago at Columbia Presbyterian Hospital they put a clot into the major artery that feeds the tumor. The tumor has shrunk to about one-third its size. It should be easier to do now.

"The second case is a routine mastectomy."

As the first patient was being wheeled into the operating room, Dr. Kendall, a chief resident surgeon, and an intern started to scrub. Because it was the first case, it would be a ten-minute scrub with Betadine, cleansing both hands to the elbows. There was a large clock over the sink to make sure that adequate time was spent scrubbing.

The operating room that Dr. Kendall was using had a glassed-in observation area with an intercom system for communication between the surgeon and the visitors. Usually the visitors were in place before the surgeon entered the room, like a theater audience. The surgeons had to be dressed properly: special boots with conductors to prevent static electricity from igniting anesthetic agents; a special cap for the head; and plastic protective goggles covered the surgeon's eyes.

As Dr. Kendall entered the amphitheater he was handed a sterile towel to dry his hands and arms. He placed his hands into a rubberized waterproof gray gown that tied in front and back. The scrub nurse held out the rubber gloves and Kendall extended his hands as the scrub nurse pulled the gloves over the cuffs of the gown.

By this time the anesthesiologist had intravenous tubing inserted into the patient's veins and a large central line placed into the right neck veins in case of a massive blood loss. An endotracheal tube had been passed through the nose, down the oral cavity, past the vocal chords, and into the main stem bronchus for oxygenation. A rubber balloon cuff on the end of the anesthesia tube was blown up to lock the tube in place and prevent aspiration of stomach contents if the patient vomited.

The resident surgeon prepped the neck and cheek area on the left side and the upper cheek was cleansed with Betadine solution. Sterile drapes were then placed around the patient's neck. Plastic compression boots that created and released pressure against the legs were hooked up to a machine to prevent clots from developing during the operation.

A Foley catheter was placed in the bladder to monitor urinary output. A tube was passed through the mouth down the esophagus to the approximate area of the heart to monitor the heartbeat. Wires were hooked up to a machine that recorded a continuous electrocardiogram. Another special device that looked like a clothespin was clamped over a fingernail to determine the oxygenation of the blood.

After Dr. Kendall and his assisting resident surgeons were completely gowned by the chief scrub nurse, he spoke to Dr. Jack Hanson, the chief surgical resident who would be across the operating table from him, assisting in the operation.

"Jack, why don't you briefly tell these visiting doctors about this patient's problem."

"OK," replied Dr. Hanson. He turned and faced the visiting doctors. "Mr. Gordon is a fifty-four-year-old white male who presented two weeks ago with a large, grapefruit-sized mass in the left neck. He was first seen in this hospital by an ENT doctor eighteen years ago with a swelling in the left tonsillar area. A tonsillectomy was done and the patient almost bled to death on the operating table. After he was discharged, the tonsillar area had to be repeatedly sutured in the emergency room because of intermittent bleeding.

"The patient was then referred to Dr. Kendall, who ordered an arteriogram to outline the blood-vessel architecture of the mass. This revealed a vascular carotid body tumor nestled at the bifurcation of the major blood vessels to the head.

"What the ear, nose and throat specialist thought was an enlarged tonsil was in reality a large vascular tumor in the neck bulging against the left tonsil area.

"Eighteen years ago, Dr. Kendall resected the tumor with substantial blood loss. The tumor recurred nine years later and was resected on three separate occasions during the next 18 years. Because of the rarity and difficulty in resecting and treating this tumor, the patient was seen in consultation in Boston, New York City, Chicago, and St. Louis. He continued to work and eventually became a Senior Vice President at one of the major aircraft companies in St. Louis.

"Mr. Gordon returned to Whitestone Hospital two weeks ago with a large recurrent tumor (the size of a grapefruit), encompassing his left middle and upper neck. The patient had diffuse involvement with the major blood vessels of the neck, including the main artery that goes to the brain, the carotid, so we decided to try a unique new experimental method to shrink the tumor.

"An invasive radiologist tried to shrink the size of the tumor by plugging the large blood vessels that fed the tumor with gel foam and liquid silastic mixed with tantalum powder. This was done in New York City at Columbia Presbyterian Medical Center. A thin plastic catheter was inserted into the patient's femoral artery in the leg and, under x-ray control, was directed to the left neck carotid artery that fed the tumor mass. Special clotting material was then passed through the tube to plug the major blood vessel to the tumor. The tumor dramatically decreased in size, making surgical removal possible.

"You can see on the x-rays over there on the view box that the patient now presents with a recurrent carotid body tumor involving the left upper neck and pharynx area extending up to the base of the skull. The bulk of the tumor occludes part of the oral cavity inside the mouth and is symptomatic.

"Work-up included bilateral angiograms of the carotid arteries to determine blood flow to the brain. The right side is clear but the left side is almost completely occluded by the tumor.

"Dr. Kendall plans to resect the entire left common carotid artery from the clavicle to the base of the skull, with the tumor. He's planning to split the mandible to get better access to the base of the skull."

While the case was being summarized for the visitors, the anesthesiologists had put the patient to sleep.

Dr. Kendall took his place on the left side of the operating table, the chief resident surgeon across from him. The chief scrub nurse, Ms. Vincent, was also opposite Dr. Kendall to hand him instruments as he worked. Kendall's head seldom moved as his eyes focused on the operative field.

The surgeon glanced over at the senior anesthesiologist and said, "OK to start?"

The reply was yes.

Matt's right forefinger went out, which was a hand signal for a scalpel that was firmly placed in his hand by Ms. Vincent. He quickly made the incision, which extended from the clavicle to the base of the skull.

"I'll use the laser," said Dr. Kendall, and she handed him the special equipment.

Using the laser and the Neomed cautery, he rapidly developed superior and inferior flaps under the skin and then sutured the flaps open to expose the anatomy around the tumor. There was little bleeding because of the use of the laser and Neomed cautery that cauterized the vessels as he worked.

He then asked for a high-powered Hall air drill to split the mandible to gain access to the major blood vessels at the base of the skull. The air drill precisely cut the bone as if it were jelly. He then isolated the major vessels by passing vascular loops around them.

Starting at the lower part of the neck, Matt ligated the left common carotid artery, one of the largest blood vessels that go to the brain, tying it quickly and then dividing it. Each small feeding blood vessel to the tumor had to be tied. He took care not to injure the large vagus nerve that sends branches to the vocal chords and heart and to the motor nerves that control the motion of the tongue, and the facial nerve. When he dissected to the base of the skull, he ligated the major artery and vein. This was extremely difficult and time consuming, because the artery was involved with the tumor.

Now with most of the blood vessels tied, the tumor shrank even more and was quickly dissected. The skin flaps were then sutured back together by the chief resident surgeon.

When the case was finished, Matt was sore and stiff from standing in one place and tired from continuous exhausting concentration. He felt good inside because he had succeeded in what he had set out to do. He had used very little blood (two units), and the operative procedure had gone well. He left the operating room and went to the doctor's lounge for coffee and to meet with the visiting doctors. They were particularly interested in learning about the embolization technique used to shrink the tumor.

One of the visitors came up to Dr. Kendall and said, "That's a pretty neat trick, that embolization technique."

"Well, it makes an inoperable case operable," he replied. "The mortality on this operation with blood loss and stroke used to be fifty percent. It's now down to less than five percent."

"Were you worried that the patient might have a stroke when you tied off that main artery to the brain?" asked another.

"Not really," replied Matt. "We checked out the vascular supply to the brain on the opposite side and it was clear."

"Do you think he might develop another recurrent tumor?"

"Who knows?" replied Matt. "We've kept him alive for eighteen years and he's continued to be a successful businessman. I know he won't get it back in his left neck because we've taken all those blood vessels out."

"Dr. Matt Kendall, Dr. Matt Kendall, ready in the operating room."

Matt broke off the conversation and walked down the hall to the operating scrub room and did a three-minute scrub for the next case. There were still a few visitors in the viewing area.

Dr. Hanson had the second patient prepped, draped, and ready for the operation. The left breast area was exposed.

"Tell our visitors about this patient, Jack."

"Mrs. Harnet is a forty-nine-year-old white female, who has had a biopsy showing an infiltrating ductal cancer of the left breast, measuring two inches in size. The cancer is directly under the nipple. Past history is significant. Her mother had breast cancer and she had a sister who died of it. Work-up for spread of her cancer is negative. At age thirty-nine, ten years ago, she was planning to have both breasts removed by another surgeon to prevent her from getting breast cancer and silicone implants put in. Unfortunately, when the first silicone implant was put in the right breast after removal of the breast tissue, the implant developed a leak followed by an overwhelming infection. The implant had to be removed. This left her with a flat, distorted chest wall.

"The surgeon who did this operation retired and the patient was then referred to Dr. Kendall for follow-up. Two weeks ago, a mammogram suggested a suspicious calcified lesion in the left breast and a biopsy revealed a classical infiltrating ductal cancer—the most common type of breast cancer.

"She and her husband explored various options with Dr. Kendall. Conservation surgery was discussed. A second opinion was also obtained. The patient chose to have the breast removed. Her comment was, 'I'd just as soon be like Twiggy since my right breast is already gone.' "

Dr. Kendall approached the operating table, put his forefinger out for the scalpel and began working. He made a long, elliptical incision over the breast from the armpit, engulfing the nipple. He quickly switched from the scalpel to the Neomed cautery. The instrument cut through the tissue and coagulated the vessels as he worked. Very few blood vessels had to be tied. It was much easier than doing surgery the old-fashioned way, cutting with a scalpel and tying hundreds of silk sutures to control the bleeding.

He cut through the fascae covering the large muscle under the breast. Starting from below, and using the cautery, the entire base of the breast was separated from the muscle.

He gave a metal right angle retractor to his second assistant, an intern, to place under the big pectoral muscle on the chest wall, exposing the large blood vessels that went to the arm. The plan was to remove lymph glands along the main vein for study, to determine whether the breast cancer had spread to the glands under the armpit.

This part of the operation required a little more finesse, clamping the small venous tributaries and tying them with silk. Care had to be taken not to injure the nerves that went to the chest wall muscles. After the glands were removed, a Hemovac suction device with tubes was then placed in the wound to suck out debris and old blood and the skin flaps were then sutured closed.

When the case was completed, Matt took a break in the doctor's lounge.

"What do you think about the new conservation methods, lumpectomy and axillary node sampling followed by x-ray treatment?" one of the visiting doctors asked.

"It's here to stay," replied Matt, "but it doesn't completely replace mastectomy. It helps the young breast cancer patient who's sexually active."

"Why did you do a mastectomy in this case?" asked another.

"The patient requested it."

"What do you think about immediate reconstruction with silicone implants?"

"If the patient requests it, I'm willing to do it. The only thing I worry about is if a complication develops or if the implant leaks. However, I'm sure that implants will be improved in the future. The market demands it. It makes the woman feel complete again. There are numerous new methods for reconstruction of the breast."

1

Lieutenant Matt Kendall looked sharp in his dress blues with gold navy pilot wings and a chest full of brightly colored battle ribbons. He had no difficulty checking out of the service at BuPers in Arlington, Virginia. The navy experience had been good. He was 19 when he volunteered for flight training, and had matured during the past four years, flying torpedo bomber planes on night missions off the decks of carriers in the Atlantic and Pacific.

If he had the choice of volunteering for naval flight duty again, he would do it. However, he'd be more selective about the type of duty and the risks involved—he discovered he didn't enjoy being shot at and would like to forget flying at night over Tokyo and being on the deck of the U.S.S. *Saratoga* when a bunch of crazy Japanese kamikaze pilots tried to sink his ship off the coast of Iwo Jima. That attack was too close for comfort and many of his shipmates and flying buddies had been killed.

If anyone was ready for the challenge of civilian life, Matt was. Young, bronzed, lean, and healthy, the ex-navy pilot was ready to go back to college to become a doctor. He was glad to be out of the service and back in the real world.

Before leaving Washington, DC, he was to pick up Becky, the beautiful navy C.P.O. to whom he was engaged. They had spent their last night together, sharing their love and vowing to remain faithful. Becky had been pretty torn up all night and wasn't happy about the separation. Matt had decided to go back to take a premed course at a small New England college, and she was to return home to Kansas City. Becky would enter the University of Iowa and Matt was worried about her. She was a traffic-stopper and would be a prime target for all the men on campus. Becky was not worried. Matt was going back to an all-male college.

He was still in his uniform when he went to pick her up at her apartment. She was in uniform and gave him a smart salute, which he returned.

"That's the last salute I'll ever get," he said. "And you're the one who should do it. You won't have any more of that nonsense when you get into civilian clothes."

"I know," said Becky. "I wonder how much I'm going to miss it. I know I'm going to miss you!" There were tears in her eyes. "Matt, please come here." He did, and pulled her close, gave her a big hug and kiss. "During these past six months you've made me come alive. I can't bear the thought of being away from you."

"Don't worry, honey, I'm going to stay in touch. I promise."

"It won't be the same," said Becky.

"I know. If all goes well, we'll get married as soon as I finish my undergraduate studies."

"That's such a long time away. You may change. I may change. I don't like it."

"I don't either. But we don't have a choice."

The cab came to pick them up for the trip to Washington National Airport. Becky cried all the way.

"Oh, God, Matt, I miss you already and you haven't even left. Why don't we just elope and forget the rest of our plans."

"I can't and I think you know why. I've got to prove to myself that I have what it takes to get into medical school. Once that's accomplished, I'll know I can take care of you for the rest of your life."

All too soon, there was an announcement over the loudspeaker: "Last call for Flight 622 to Kansas City."

Becky kissed Matt, her cheeks warm and wet against his. She ran to the plane and when she got to the top of the ramp she turned, waved once, and disappeared inside. Matt took a deep breath, blinked back his own tears, and walked away.

When he arrived in Connecticut, he enrolled at Trinity College, a small school with an excellent reputation for preparing students for medicine. His college tuition would be paid for by the G.I. Bill. He knew the adjustment to civilian life would not be an easy one. He had grown accustomed to being in the fast track as a navy pilot, and living in a high-priced apartment on Connecticut Avenue in Washington, DC. He had received fat monthly paychecks for hazardous flying duty, and enjoyed flying expensive airplanes around the country. Now, he would have an abrupt change in his lifestyle, living at home and commuting by bus to the college campus.

Matt was worried about the new struggle he faced, competing against younger classmates from prep schools and high schools. Most of the freshmen students had not been in the service and were accustomed to concentrated study habits. He would have to learn how to study all over again. The premed course he had signed up for was considered the toughest major at the college.

His first week of classes was rough. He felt overwhelmed. The bad news was that the professors didn't look friendly and the workload was formidable. The good news was that the professors who were teaching the courses were well trained and highly qualified.

He would remember his first day in biology class forever. Professor Somerset was a portly, well-dressed gentleman who, despite his bow tie, looked tougher than a marine master sergeant. There were 60 ambitious first-year students in his class and they all wanted to be doctors. Some of them were sons of doctors or dentists. Others, like Matt, were former G.I.s.

Professor Somerset spoke to the class. "Gentlemen, look around you. There are sixty of you in my class. You are all intelligent students, or you wouldn't be here. However, the health of our country and finding solutions to many challenges in medicine requires that only the best of you become doctors. What that means is that twenty of you will be given grades above eighty and will receive a letter of recommendation to go on to medical school. Ten will receive grades above seventy and they will receive letters of recommendation for dental school. The rest of you will either drop out of the premed major or will seek other fields of endeavor with my blessing. You will have two major examinations in this course; the midterm and the final. There will also be four unannounced one-hour quizzes."

With that announcement, there was a big groan from the students.

"That's to keep you alert at all times," he said. "A doctor deals with life-and-death decisions and a good doctor's life is dedicated to the public and to continuing his own education. He can never tell when he will be called on in an emergency."

When the class finished, Matt and a few students got together at the college canteen. "Boy, it's going to be cutthroat," said one of the students.

"Does anyone have a book on Professor Somerset?"

"The frat houses have his old exams, but he never repeats the same questions. He's wise to the students."

"How are we going to beat him, then?"

"At his own game," said Matt. "Study hard, and hope for the best."

As he went home, he thought the biology course was going to be a bitch. But it was crucial to his plans for the future. He studied deep into the night, burning the midnight oil for the next four weeks. He worked harder than he had for years.

On a Monday morning after a big football weekend, the students entered the biology classroom, and the shades were drawn over the blackboard. The time had arrived.

Somerset came in, handed out paper, pulled the shades up, and on the blackboard was the first unannounced quiz. It was a shocker, for it was not a multiple choice exam. All the answers had to be in essay form. Some of the questions were impossible to answer directly—they weren't based on memory. You had to put things together to get the answer. In other words, you had to think.

Before Matt finished the exam he had palpitations, a cold sweat, and he felt a good case of diarrhea coming on. He was sure he had flunked the quiz, and when the grades were posted, he had. He had scored a 50. The professor even had the audacity to write on the bottom of his paper, "*Arbeiten schwer.*" Matt had to get a German dictionary to find out what it meant. It was a German term that meant "work hard." But Somerset didn't stop there. He posted everyone's grades on the wall for everyone to see, starting with the highest grades on top. Matt was tenth from the bottom. He was pissed off! All that work for nothing!

He wasn't alone. Most of the returning veterans were right there on the bottom of the list with him and they were in a panic. Three of the young prep school squirts in the class had gotten A's and one scored a 97.

"We ought to bump that guy off," said one of the veterans. "It would mean one less pre-med to beat."

Damn! What a disaster, thought Matt. Something drastic had to be done.

The veterans were depressed. They decided to go over the hill to a beer joint and discuss their rude awakening. "It looks like we may end up as truck drivers," one said.

"In some way, we're going to have to beat Professor Somerset."

"How are we going to do that?" asked Norman, a former infantry captain.

"We're going to make book on him. We'll study together to compare class notes and analyze his exams. If we want to survive and make the grade, we'll forget the girls and the football games. We've got one shot at getting into medical school and that means getting our grades into the top twenty."

"Why don't we all just quit and take some gut courses that will prepare us to be brokers," said Beckwith, one of the veterans. "We can sit on our asses and make a lot of dough."

"You have to be a crook to be successful in that field," said Norman. "Besides, you'll never get any satisfaction out of life unless you put something worthwhile back into it. I didn't fight in the infantry to come back and become a broker."

Matt, Norman and the other two veterans went to work. They quizzed each other weekly and studied in the library till closing.

The second exam came all too soon. All four thought they had done better. When the grades were posted, they had raised their grades from 50 to 75 and were in the middle of the class. The result encouraged them to work harder. They celebrated with pizza and a few beers.

The teamwork of the four veterans eventually paid off. Matt received a final grade of 88 and his buddies were all in the 80s. He finished fifth in his class in the biology course and had a shot at medical school. He decided to go to summer school and take some courses to catch up with the premed students who had not served in the armed forces. He hoped to get additional credits to graduate sooner. Two of the courses were chemistry: qualitative and quantitative analysis.

One major hurdle remained before completing undergraduate premed studies: organic chemistry. This one was an ass-buster. It was taught by Professor Vernon Kringle, the department head, and it dealt with chemical compounds and how they're formed. Students had to memorize hundreds of formulas and the methods of making chemical compounds.

One week before the final exam, the light bulb went on in Matt's brain and he really cracked the exam. He got an A in the course. His buddies did well also.

Medical schools were flooded with applications at that time, so Matt decided to take an additional year of postgraduate education and was accepted at Columbia University in New York for a master's degree in biology. He was all set to go, but just prior to Christmas vacation of his senior year, as he was picking up his books at the chemistry building, he ran into the head of the Chemistry Department, Professor Kringle.

"Matt, what are you planning to do next year?" he asked.

"I'm going to New York to attend Columbia University. I'm going for my Master's in biology."

"I thought you wanted to be a doctor of medicine?"

"I do," said Matt, "but I don't think I have a chance with so many people applying to medical school."

"Did you take the MedCats?"

"Yes."

"Do you know how you did on them?"

"No, but they didn't seem to be too tough."

"How old are you?"

"Twenty-five."

"You should go to medical school now."

"It's too late," said Matt, "All the classes are filled."

"We'll see about that. Come into my office."

When they got into Professor Kringle's office, he told his secretary to get one of the junior professors to take his next class. He called the MedCat Center to get Matt's grades.

"Matt, you did well on your MedCats. Who is your faculty advisor?"

"Professor Wells."

"I can't believe this. Didn't he talk to you?"

"No. What should I do?"

"I'll take care of it. I'm going to make some phone calls."

The next day he received a call from Dr. Kringle's office and he went to see him.

"You're going to visit some medical schools next week," said Professor Kringle. "We're going to get you into next year's class."

"I have to take my final exams next week. I can't go."

"Don't worry about that. I'll talk to your professors."

Matt took a train to Rochester, New York; St. Louis, Missouri; Philadelphia, Pennsylvania; and New Haven, Connecticut. He met the deans of four medical schools and had good interviews with all of them.

The following week, he received letters of acceptance from all four. He went to see Professor Kringle and asked him which one he should attend.

"Which one did you like?" he asked.

"I was impressed by the dean at the University of Rochester Medical

School, George H. Wilson. I understand that he won the Nobel Prize in medicine."

"That's right," said Professor Kringle. "Then you should go there and make some impressions of your own."

Matt was ecstatic. He had gotten into medical school and, if he studied hard, he would realize his dream. He would become a doctor of medicine.

He had worked hard after getting out of the Navy Air Corps. Four years in the navy had delayed his time clock and he still felt like he was trying to catch up. He took five courses each semester and went to two summer school sessions, making up a whole year of college. His time spent in the service was not completely wasted. He had seen the world, seen it at war, and had grown up in it. The war had given him Rebecca.

She corresponded with him regularly, flooding his mailbox with letters.

They finally set the date to get married. Matt's father was furious. He was opposed to the marriage. He felt that if Matt got married he wouldn't go on with his education. A battle royal developed. Finally his father told him that he would be disowned. It was not the first time threats had been passed between them.

Becky was also not happy about Matt becoming a doctor. The educational process was long, the financial return distant. She didn't like the idea that she would have to work while he went to school.

No one from Matt's family was coming to the wedding because of his father's decree. Still, 250 invitations were sent out and many of his navy flying buddies planned to attend.

Chuck Strong was to be the best man and Domkowski, who was now a Lieutenant Commander flying in the navy, would be one of the ushers. Becky had selected her bridesmaids and had bought her wedding gown. It was to be a formal wedding with white tie and tails followed by a large reception at the local country club. They were planning to spend their honeymoon in Washington, DC, where they met.

One week before the wedding Matt took a plane to Kansas City and Becky met him at the airport. She was still as pretty as he had remembered her. She gave him a big hug and kiss and told him how much she had missed him.

"We've got a lot of things to talk about," said Rebecca. "I'm so happy."

"I know," replied Matt. "So am I."

Becky came to the point. She looked him straight in the eyes and said, "Are you sure you want to go to medical school?"

"Of course," he said. "I'm as sure of that as I am of marrying you."

She smiled and looked down. "It's going to be a long struggle and I want to have at least two or three children."

"I know. We'll have to postpone some of our plans."

"Not all of them, I hope."

"What are our plans for tonight?"

"We're having a dinner party at my house."

"Are we going to get to be alone?"

"Of course we are."

That plan didn't materialize. There were 75 guests whom Becky and her parents had invited to attend the party. Most of them were family friends and men and women who had gone to college with her. There were a few young lawyers and dentists in the crowd. They were all interested in meeting the former pilot from New England who Becky had picked for her husband.

There was a young lawyer who was particularly attentive to Becky. Matt had not anticipated this type of an evening. There was something chaotic in the air. He could feel it. The party finally broke up around 2 A.M.

After all the guests had left, they sat down on the living room sofa. "Becky, I can hardly wait until we'll be spending all our time together."

"I know," she said, as she drew close and kissed him. She had full, sensuous lips and she moved to him so he slid his hands around her waist. But when he started to caress her, she pushed him away.

"I'm saving that part for our wedding night."

"You've got to be kidding. Listen, we've been apart for a long time, have you forgotten who I am? I'm not exactly a stranger."

"Of course you're not. It's been almost two years since we've gotten together and there's a lot of talking and catching up to do. I have to get to know you all over again."

So it was back to puppy love and hand-holding for Matt. Rebecca had drawn the line. Yes, she responded to his kisses. Yes, she was right there. But that was as far as she was willing to go.

It was a frustrating night for him. Oh hell, he thought, in ten days we'll be married. In the meantime, it's back to the cold showers. Wouldn't be the first time, but hopefully it could be the last.

"Matt, tomorrow you and I have to go over the final plans for the wedding," said Becky. "Pick me up and we'll have breakfast together."

"OK."

The next morning he picked her up at her home. Her father, a dentist, and her mother were there to greet him. While he waited for Becky, her dad took him into the den and Matt thought, here we go.

"How's the budding doctor doing?" asked Dr. Harper.

"Well, I've gotten into medical school, and that's half the battle," said Matt.

"That's only the beginning," said Dr. Harper. "Are you planning to specialize or be a general practitioner? How do you plan to pay for your education?"

"I have the G.I. Bill of Rights. That will pay for five years of my education."

And then the shoe dropped. "How do you plan to support my daughter?"

"It'll be a struggle, but we'll survive."

"Love doesn't put food on the table. How old are you?"

"Twenty-five," he replied. He was determined not to drop his self-assurance.

"That's not very young to be starting medical school. Why don't you consider going into some other field that has a shorter training period? Why don't you become a dentist?"

"Because I want to be a real doctor."

"If I were you, I'd give it some thought," said Dr. Harper. "Look at me, a relatively short training education, eight years to be exact. Now I have a dental practice that I have difficulty keeping up with. I've got more money than I know what to do with. It's pretty much a cash business. When you finish dental school you could come into my office."

"Don't you get bored working in the mouth all the time?" asked Matt.

"Not really, particularly when I take the week's receipts to the bank," the dentist smiled.

With that remark, Dr. Harper left the room and drove away in his touring Cadillac to go to work in downtown Kansas City.

Matt gave his comments some serious thought as Becky got into his rental car and he drove to a restaurant for breakfast. Rebecca was still a very vivacious, beautiful woman and her choice of clothing was exquisite. He began to wonder how he would be able to afford her clothes. Maybe her father was right.

"What did you and my dad talk about?" asked Becky.

"My future and yours."

"Did he tell you that he had a job for you if you want it?"

"No, in fact he didn't. He alluded to the possibility of working side by side with him, as a dentist, however."

"I don't want your pride hurt, but Daddy said that a vice president of one of the large pharmaceutical houses in the city has a great job opening. You'd be trained in sales and cover this area of the country. We wouldn't have any financial worries."

"I don't want to be a pharmaceutical salesman. It would put me on the sidelines and I'd always wonder what it would have been like to be in the game. This is important for me. And us."

The dialogue concerning the long training period to become a doctor continued throughout the next couple days.

"I worked hard in undergraduate school so I could go to medical school. I don't plan to throw all that effort away."

"Well, can you see my point of view?" asked Becky.

"Yes I can," said Matt. "You're apprehensive about marrying me and not having a big initial income."

"Yes, I am. But I feel I still love you."

"Have you been dating out here, while I was in the East?"

"Yes."

"Is there anyone in particular?"

"Not really. But that lawyer you commented about has been quite attentive."

"No doubt," said Matt sarcastically.

Suddenly Becky began to cry. "Oh, Matt, we had it so good in Washington when you were flying. Why didn't we get married then and you could have stayed in the navy?"

"I'd probably be dead by now flying those jets off the carriers at night. And you know that part of my life ended with the war. Now speak your heart. What do you want to do, Becky?"

"I need more time to think," she said. "I want to wait. I'm going to call off the wedding." She had tears in her eyes.

"That's your choice," said Matt. "We'll have to send telegrams out to all our friends who are planning to come to the wedding."

"My Dad said he'd take care of that. Oh, Matt, I'm so sorry," said Becky.

"Not as sorry as I am."

The next morning he took a plane to St. Louis. Chuck Strong was at Lambert Field to meet him and Molly, his wife, was with him.

"What happened?" asked Chuck.

"Becky didn't want to marry a guy who would be going to school for the rest of his life just to become a doctor."

"Is it finished?" asked Chuck.

"As far as I'm concerned it is, and I don't want to discuss it any further."

2

FOR MATT KENDALL, going from undergraduate college to medical school was like flying a Piper Cub airplane with a maximum speed of 70 miles an hour and then stepping into the cockpit of a jet for the first time.

In the late 1940s, the prestige of doctors was unsurpassed in the United States. Medical ethics were regarded as impeccable and the profession was looked at with admiration by the public. There was no such thing as suing a doctor for malpractice and most doctors did not have malpractice insurance. Doctors were placed on a pedestal the same way clerics, judges, and magistrates were. This made the profession a sought-after trade by the veterans of World War II; they thought it would be a good way to earn a living and be looked up to in their community.

There were 70 members in Matt's medical school class and many of the students wore the gold Phi Beta Kappa key. The students were told by the faculty that the whole class could have been filled with Phi Beta Kappas but the admissions committee wanted to have a diverse student body that excelled not only in academics, but in other fields of endeavor. Approximately 15 members of the class had served in the armed services during World War II.

The day before orientation began, Matt went to the bookstore to buy the medical books for his classes. He was surprised by their size and cost: *Gray's Anatomy, Best and Taylor Physiology, Goodman and Gilman Pharmacology*, and *Ackerman's Pathology*. Just carrying those books home delivered a message: Get ready for the academic ordeal of your life.

One of the first things he had to do was find a place to live. There was no dormitory housing for medical students, so he had to look for a room within walking distance of the hospital. He had been given a list of nearby rooming houses by the medical school. After searching, he found a three-family house that had a loft. He would share the space with two younger medical students; one from Cornell and the other from Hobart. The price was reasonable and the woman who took care of the place kept it clean.

Part of the first day's festivities at medical school was a get-together with the faculty and a talk given to the entering freshman class by the Associate Dean. It was an unexpected ego boost.

"You are a highly select group of students. Each year the number of medical school applicants continues to grow. Some of you have achieved excellence in academics beyond the undergraduate years and have already contributed to medical research. Others have had their education delayed by the war. Each of you has been hand-picked by the faculty and are expected to graduate with honors.

"No matter what your past achievements have been, however, you will all be starting out as equals in the endeavor to become a doctor of medicine. Not all your courses will be stimulating or challenging. Some of you may think they're boring. However, they should be considered building blocks, helping you learn fundamentals about the human body. As you continue to study medicine and become wiser, you will learn that the human body is the most complex organism that lives on this earth. All of you will get to know the stress and pressure that a doctor has to endure. You will be taught how to think like a doctor and to adopt a professional demeanor that can be easily recognized by the public. A good doctor is a humble doctor who is committed to put the care of his patients first. The constant changes in medicine—sophistication of new diagnostic techniques and instrumentation, and new treatment methods—require that you continue to study to maintain your skills for the rest of your life.

"Your first year, you will learn about anatomy, histology, physiology, and biochemistry. In your second year you will study pharmacology and physical diagnosis. You will be introduced to the ravages of disease when you study pathology.

"Medical students complain about the basic sciences. They often comment that basic sciences are too time-consuming and unnecessary. You will find, sooner or later, that the application of the information gained from the basic sciences will determine whether you become a mediocre, good, or excellent doctor.

"The art and practice of medicine and surgery changes every day and the challenges can be overwhelming. Some of you will become general practitioners. Others will become specialists. But all of you who graduate from this medical school will remain students and teachers for the rest of your lives.

"One last comment: All of us on the staff of the medical school are extremely happy to have you with us and are here to teach you. In order to accomplish this we must communicate. If we fail, you fail. We don't want that to happen. Don't hesitate to ask questions. Good luck to all of you."

The next day, medical school began.

The anatomy class was taught by Dr. Charles Tobias, an excellent teacher. There were lectures in the course, but what it really boiled down to was spending hours dissecting a human body and trying to recognize and memorize all the numerous different parts.

Gross anatomy is of such a tremendous scope that there is no way a freshman medical student can hope to gain a complete practical knowledge of all phases of the structure of the human body. The aim for the student in the dissecting room was to gain sufficient anatomical understanding so that knowledge could later be integrated and applied.

The first day of dissection, the students were reminded by the professors that the body they were working on was once a human being and that they should treat that body with respect within the context of their work.

With modern methods of embalming and preservation, decay is not a factor and most bodies were in excellent shape. A sharp scalpel, blunt pointed forceps, and a pair of medium-sized scissors were used in the dissection. The professor and his assistants would circulate around the dissecting tables to aid in recognizing difficult anatomical areas.

Matt's first problem was trying to recognize and memorize all the anatomical names of the body parts he had to dissect. Fortunately, there were three other students dissecting the same body and together they constantly reviewed the texts and tested each other.

Every three or four weeks, they had a laboratory anatomy quiz. Numbers with arrows were placed on anatomical structures and the students would walk from station to station and be given a short time to identify the structure. Not all the bodies were the same and not all bodies were dissected as well as others. There were times when Matt felt his brain was being bombarded with more irrelevant scientific data than it could possibly assimilate.

Histology, a branch of anatomy that deals with the minute structure of the cells and tissues, was taken at the same time as the anatomy course. Boxes of microscopic slides were handed out to each student showing what skin, heart muscle, liver tissue, breast tissue, and kidneys looked like. Being able to look at these various tissues under the microscope and recognize their proper anatomical site was not simple. Learning to use the microscope properly was an important and difficult part of the first year. Many hours were spent in the histology laboratory.

The second semester of Matt's first year brought him into physiology. It was defined by one of his professors as the study of living matter and the way it functions as cells, tissues, and organs. He was also told that it combined many disciplines in a laboratory setting. Matt didn't care how it was defined—to him it meant going back to work in the laboratory using cats, dogs, frogs, and turtles to help understand just how a body functions.

He learned that many of the anatomical structures of animals were similar to humans. One of the first experiments he performed was to study how the heartbeat works. A live turtle heart was exposed, heat was applied to a specific area, and the heartbeat increased. In contrast, placing cold over the same area would decrease the heart rate. Matt discovered that there is a sino-auricular area (S. A. node) and an auricular venticular area (A. V. node) in the turtle's heart that controlled its beat and this was true in the human heart as well.

Occasionally, during the second semester, the class would listen to a lecture by a practicing physician, who would point out the application of the basic science course in the diagnosis and treatment of a specific patient. These lectures were usually the most stimulating and commanded the students' closest attention. Finally there was a nexus between all the basic sciences, all that rote memorization, and the functioning of the human body. Matt was galvanized by the power of applied medicine and as he bent over his notes each night, he could hardly wait to be in a hospital where he could take care of patients.

Before a medical student becomes a doctor he must see what happens to the human body when illness destroys it. The medical student is first introduced to the basic study of disease, pathology, in the second year of training.

When a patient dies in the hospital, how that patient's diagnosis was established and how the patient was treated comes under close scrutiny. Each medical specialty has a weekly morbidity and mortality conference to discuss complications and deaths within their department. If a death occurs, the results of the autopsy are crucial to understanding the cause.

The pathology course at the university was taught by Dr. George H. Wilson, the dean of the medical school. It was considered the most important course students would take during their four years of study.

George H. Wilson was a tall, distinguished, gray-haired gentleman with a kind smile and an unassuming grace. He wore half glasses that he peered over and, when he set his gaze on you, his eyes had a deep, penetrating effect. To describe his appearance simply would be difficult. When he spoke, his words were well chosen. When he taught, he was deliberate and specific. One got the feeling there was a great depth and an unlimited strength of intelligence within this man. If one were to select one word to describe Dr. George Wilson, it would be "awesome." Matt and his medical school classmates were first introduced to Dean Wilson in the amphitheater of the autopsy room.

In this room the recently deceased body is placed on a metal table and dissected by the pathologist to determine the cause of death. Tissues are taken and preserved for study under the microscope.

Where technique is concerned, pathologists will never be confused with plastic surgeons. The dead body is impersonalized by long, crude knives as the pathologist makes a generous, Y-shaped incision through the chest and the entire length of the abdomen to gain access to the organs.

Sometimes the cause of death is quite evident. If the chest or abdomen is full of blood, death was probably quick from internal hemorrhage. By contrast, the ravages of disease can be seen when multiple organ systems are involved with cancer that has spread throughout the body.

It is also in the autopsy room that the medical student realizes there is something else about life and dying other than the aging process. The stress of everyday living has a profound effect on the human body and can cause the early demise of the host. Death can be as quick as blowing out a candle, and the wind of death can be excessive use of alcohol or drugs, acute stress, heart attack, or failure of the immune system.

Dr. Wilson stood before the class one day to demonstrate the gross causes of death of four patients. Human tissue specimens in separate silver trays were on the autopsy table. A resident pathologist, dressed in his white uniform, stood before the group and gave a brief history of each case and then Dr. Wilson demonstrated the findings seen in the tissues.

"Dr. Northgate, we'll start with the first tray."

Dr. Northgate faced the group and spoke in a loud, clear voice. "Claudia M. was a nine-year-old female living in a nearby farm community who had been troubled with frequent bouts of sore throats and upper respiratory infections. She had poor dental hygiene and had a recent tooth extraction. She developed the sudden onset of swelling under the jaw with an inability to swallow and difficulty breathing. Her father and mother both worked, and when her mother got home from work, she noticed her daughter had a high fever and chills and was having trouble breathing. The girl was driven thirty miles to the hospital ER. On arrival she couldn't breathe and had an obvious respiratory obstruction and a tracheostomy was done. High doses of intravenous penicillin were given. She died two hours after admission to the ER."

Dr. Wilson put on rubber gloves and lifted the neck contents out of the tray. He then spoke in a loud voice.

"This unfortunate case shows how an overwhelming undetected infection in the head and neck area can be fatal. This young child had a rapidly spreading cellulitis in the area under the tongue and jaw, forming a large abscess that obstructed her airway and caused her death." As he spoke he cut open the larynx to demonstrate a large pocket containing a white creamy pus.

"This condition is called Ludwig's angina," said Dr. Wilson. "It's a diffuse purulent inflammation of the floor of the mouth spreading to the soft tissues of the upper neck where edema and swelling can obstruct the airway. If it's not recognized early, it can cause death. This can be due to tooth extractions, tonsillar abscess, or fractures of the mandible. Are there any questions?"

One of the students raised his hand and spoke up. "Does the infection always stay in the neck?"

"No," replied Dr. Wilson, as he picked up the lungs on the tray. "She has what we call metastatic sepsis," he said, as he cut through one of the lungs, showing a lung abscess. "I'm sure she had aspiration pneumonia also. The bacterial pus in her throat spread to her lungs. Dr. Northgate will go on to the next case. Present the history for tray C," said Dr. Wilson.

"Malcolm H. is a forty-nine-year-old male farmer who contracted tuberculosis at the age of thirty-one by drinking unpasteurized milk. At that time he was placed in a TB sanitarium and was discharged three years later, improved. He was a heavy smoker and had chronic lung problems. During the past five years he was also a heavy drinker. He was admitted to the hospital three weeks ago, coughing up blood and was seen by the chest surgeons. He developed a broncho-pleural fistula, which is an opening between the lung and bronchus in the lungs, and an empyema, or abscess of his lung. Surgeons were called in for consultation and a tube to drain the pus out of his chest was put in place. However, he continued to bleed and drain pus from the drainage site. Replacement blood was given and he seemed to be doing well, except for excessive coughing. Two nights ago he had a bad coughing spell and ruptured a bleb in his opposite lung. He developed a tension pneumothorax (an air leak within the chest cavity) and the air in the closed space of the chest compressed the remaining lung. He died suddenly."

Dr. Wilson picked up the lungs, showing a large pus-like cavity. There was very little healthy lung tissue left. He found another hard nodule next to the abscess and cut through the tissue with a large knife. He looked over his half glasses, peered out at the class and fixed his stare on one of the students.

"What do you think this hard white tissue is, Mr. Stern?"

"It's probably related to his TB," he replied. "Possibly a tubercular granuloma."

"That's a possibility, but in this case you're wrong," said Dr. Wilson. "This is a lung cancer. This man has tuberculosis *and* lung cancer. Fortunately, we are seeing less TB these days. But this demonstrates that you can have more than one disease at a time.

"We'll go to tray D next, Dr. Northgate. But first, I want to ask the class some questions. How many have heard of a strep infection? Raise your hands."

Almost the entire class raised their hands. Matt remembered when he was four years old he was put to bed for four months because his doctor thought he had scarlet fever caused by a strep infection. At that time there were no antibiotics available; bed rest was the treatment. Dr. Wilson looked at the class and directed a question to Matt.

"What is one of the biggest risks when you get a strep infection, Mr. Kendall?"

He remembered his mother had told him they had to worry about his heart. "I think you can get an infection in the heart."

"That's right, and we have a case to show you where that happened," replied Dr. Wilson. "We'll go to tray E. Give a brief history to the students, Dr. Northgate."

"Sam M. is a thirty-eight-year-old male who developed the sudden onset of high fever, heart murmurs, and petechiae in the fingers, which are little blood spots under the fingernails. His health problem was not immediately recognized but he became weak and stopped going to work and was finally seen by a physician who sent him to a heart specialist. He was admitted to the hospital as an emergency and was started on massive doses of penicillin. Blood cultures were positive for streptococcus infection. On his third day in the hospital he tossed an embolism to his brain and died suddenly."

While Dr. Northgate was talking, Dr. Wilson took a scissors and opened the heart for the students to see. "This is the mitral valve of the heart," he said. "Notice there are numerous small berrylike vegetations on the valve. The aortic valve shows the same thing, obviously caused by the strep infection. This is where the embolis to the brain came from. A piece broke off the valve and went to a vital structure in the brain. Are there any questions?"

A student in the front row raised his hand.

"Yes?"

"When you get subacute bacterial endocarditis, are any other organs involved?" he asked.

"Good question. You can get an enlarged spleen." He picked up a spleen three times its normal size. "You can also get an infarction of the kidney or a liver or brain abscess.

"We'll do one more case," said Dr. Wilson. "Dr. Northgate, give a brief history about that unfortunate GYN case. Tray G."

"June D., is a nineteen-year-old black girl who was brought into the ER two nights ago with acute abdominal pain, a temperature of 105 degrees and vaginal bleeding. Past history is significant in that this patient was a known prostitute and had a criminal record.

"A male brought her in at 4:00 A.M. and left the ER. A phone call later revealed that an abortion had been attempted with a coat hanger during the preceding week.

"On admission to the ER, it was felt the patient was in septic shock. Blood cultures were drawn to see if bacteria had gotten into her bloodstream and she was started on high doses of intravenous penicillin. She had a markedly elevated white blood count of 28,000 and yellow jaundice with blood changes causing black and blue bruises all over her body.

"X-rays of the abdomen revealed air in her belly under the diaphragm. This suggested that when the coat hanger was used in the attempted abortion, the uterus or bowel was perforated and the bacterial organisms and air got into the abdominal cavity. The patient died two hours after admission to the ER."

Dr. Wilson picked up the tray containing the pelvic organs and spoke up. "This unfortunate female had non-professional help concerning her pregnancy. She was involved with a criminal abortion. I'm now demonstrating the hole or tear through the uterus into the abdominal cavity. There's also a hole in the small bowel. There's fecal contamination of the abdominal cavity. This was either self-inflicted or, as stated, by an accessory using a coat hanger. Her blood cultures were all positive. Her blood pressure disappeared in septic shock and her kidneys shut down. All her pelvic organs became involved with an overwhelming infection that killed her."

The class, which to that point had shown no discomfort, shifted in their chairs uneasily. Dr. Wilson looked up. "Good," he said. "You should feel upset! When you cease to be fazed by the senseless loss of a human life, you should think about another profession!"

The second-year medical students eventually had direct contact with George H. Wilson eyeball to eyeball. Every Friday morning the students placed their chairs in a circle around his desk. Dean Wilson carried a small notebook with pictures of all the students. He would flip through that notebook and call on one of the students to sit in a chair facing his desk; this seat was called "the pit."

The apprehension before Friday's class was overwhelming. There were frequent last-minute visits to the bathroom, and more than a few pale faces. Some had cold sweats. Others frantically searched through their notes for a quick glance at a subject they might be quizzed about.

Once the dean walked into the class, a student would be called to take his place in the pit and the interrogation would begin.

In the moment before the selection, there was a thin, brittle silence as he flipped through the pages of his notebook. Some of the early questions directed to the student were easy, an attempt to get the student to relax. The dean's ability to take a subject and demonstrate the most important aspects through questions was apparent each time he grilled someone in the pit. He would often comment about the student's answers and make additions that summarized the material. If a student seemed to be getting all the answers correct, he would inject a few tougher questions.

Performing in "the pit" couldn't be faked. Dean Wilson's oral exam was at times like interrogation, at others like having a lively chat. Wilson explored and probed the corridors of his students' minds like he might any bodily part, investigating until he discovered its nature and function.

In one class they had cultured the bacteria taken from under their fingernails and grew them out in Petri dishes. After you looked at all those different wiggly life forms under the microscope, you had no desire to stick your fingers in your mouth—a strong deterrent to the nail-biting Dean Wilson's cross-examination caused.

On a mid-semester Friday morning, Dean Wilson called out, "Mr. Matt Kendall, front and center."

Matt took his seat in front of Dr. Wilson. He noticed his heart rate had increased as he looked up at the distinguished dean.

The dean spoke up as he peered over his half glasses at Matt. "Mr. Kendall, you've been in the autopsy room and laboratory many times now. What sort of cases have you been impressed with?"

"I've been impressed with the frequency of heart and cancer cases," he replied.

"Good," said Dean Wilson. "Perhaps we'll talk a little bit about cancer today and maybe later about the heart. How would you define cancer?"

Matt drew a blank. Then perspiration broke out on his brow. He hesitated and finally blurted out, "I'll give it a try. I think a lot of people are trying to find out just what cancer is. The term is derived from the Greek word karkinos, or crab. It was named by Hippocrates because of the pincer-like projections he noticed when examining women with breast cancer."

A smile came to Dean Wilson's face. "I'm delighted somebody is reading about the history of medicine. However, that answer is not quite what I had in mind."

Some of Matt's classmates giggled in the background.

"Could you elaborate?" asked the dean. "Just what is a cancer cell?"

There was a long pause as Matt tried to think.

"Well," he replied, "a cancer cell is a cell that has gone haywire. It's a new growth or abnormal mass of tissue that preys on the host. I believe it is capable of local invasion and can spread to distant anatomical sites."

"Let's be a little bit more specific," said the dean. "Just what does a cancer cell look like under the microscope?"

Matt thought for a minute. He and two other students had talked about that. He finally spoke up. "The cancer cell and the nuclei within the center of the cell show variations in size and shape. The cells can appear abnormal. They can be many times larger than their neighbors or may be small and appear premature."

"I'll accept that," said the dean.

Suddenly Matt felt he may have gotten the answer correct and became slightly exhilarated. He wanted to get at least a few answers correct in front of his classmates.

"How do you tell the difference between a benign or malignant tumor?" asked the dean. "Are there any similarities?"

He's getting me deeper into the pit. How am I going to answer this one? A lot of tumors—benign or malignant—looked the same to me. In fact, his fellow students had talked to him about that one too!

"I suppose they both have blood vessels to feed the growing abnormal tissue, and something to support it."

"What is that something to support it?" asked the dean. "How do you keep that new uncontrolled abnormal tissue and blood vessels together?"

"I don't know," he replied, with as much dignity as he could muster.

"What do you see around those abnormal cells and blood vessels under the microscope?" asked the dean.

"I suppose you can see some fat and connective tissue."

"It is connective tissue," said the dean. "Just a few more questions."

Matt felt twinges of pain in his stomach. He didn't like being in "the pit" and he knew his luck would run out. He was afraid he might get diarrhea and have to run out to the bathroom if the questioning continued much longer.

"What does it mean when a pathologist says the cells of a tumor are poorly differentiated when he's looking under the microscope?"

"It means the cells and the nuclei within the cells are all different sizes and shapes. Some are larger than their neighbors and others are extremely small and primitive-appearing."

"What does the term well-differentiated tumor mean?

"It means the tumor is composed of cells resembling the normal cells of the tissue. They all look healthy and the same."

"Can a malignant tumor be well differentiated or undifferentiated?"

Matt drew a blank. He had reached bottom. He was getting nervous and really sweating. "I'm certain I don't know that answer," he replied.

There it was, another smile on Dean Wilson's face.

"Well, a malignant tumor can be both," said Dean Wilson. "Most benign tumors are well differentiated. Malignant tumors can be well differentiated or undifferentiated."

Matt felt he had run out of gas. That sponge in his skull wasn't working any more. He wished the inquisition would stop. He was getting embarrassed in front of his classmates.

"There's a specimen up here on the table by my desk in the tray," said the dean. "I want you to look at it and tell me what you think it might be."

Here's the bomb, he thought. He walked up to the table. There was a big grapefruit-like piece of meat with a lot of yellow fatty tissue around it. He had no idea what it might be.

"You can put some gloves on and feel it," said Dean Wilson. "Go ahead."

Matt put the big thick yellow gloves on as his classmates smiled. The specimen was semisoft and mushy and had some skin attached. He had no idea what it was. Rather than give the wrong answer, he replied, "I have no idea what this tissue is. I'd ask for a consult." There was a burst of laughter from the class.

The dean was disturbed and snapped his head around. He looked up over his half glasses at the students. His eyes had a message. It was quite clear. The class realized their mistake. Suddenly there was silence.

"Well," said the dean. "I'm going to pass out some pieces of paper that I want you all to write on. You're to come up, and look and feel this specimen. First, write your name on the paper. Second, write down what organ or tissue it is. Third, write down what you think the pathology is. We'll see just how many of you can get the correct answer!"

When they went back to class the next week they were told that no one had gotten the correct answer. The dean had gotten his point across. It was not to be their last lesson in humility.

"The pit" truly was an equalizer!

3

NEAR THE END of his second year, Matt and his classmates were introduced to laboratory procedures. They were taught how to do vein punctures to draw blood and start intravenous feedings; obtain urine samples for microscopic examination; pass Levine tubes to empty the stomach or decompress the stomach prior to surgery; do bleeding and clotting times from a finger stick.

The guinea pigs for teaching students how to draw blood were fellow classmates. A tourniquet would be put on the classmate's arm and then one's partner would slide the needle directly into a vein. Some students were better than others in obtaining samples, and a few passed out at the sight of needles.

The students were also taught how to determine blood types and to do white blood counts to tell if an infection was present.

They were shown how to check the prostate of the male and the vagina and cervix of the female. The importance of a rectal exam was also demonstrated. They were also taught to take a small glove sample of stool, which could then be checked for occult blood and, if blood was present, a proctosigmoidoscopy could be done to help determine where the blood was coming from. A tube with a light (sigmoidoscope) could be put in the rectum and into the lower bowel to investigate and visualize abnormalities.

Blood cultures, throat cultures, urine cultures—all of these basic tests were taught to track the source of infection. Skin tests were also demonstrated to determine allergies. Oral glucose tolerance and intravenous glucose tolerance tests were taught to see if a patient was diabetic.

Most students were eager to get into their third year so that they could start their clinical clerkships and begin seeing patients. The students would rotate in six- to eight-week shifts, hopping from medicine to surgery to pediatrics to obstetrics and gynecology, then on to urology, orthopedics, and neurosurgery. Usually an intern would be assigned to work with three or four medical students, instructing them in how to take a history and perform a good physical examination.

The longest rotations were spent on the general surgical service and the medical service, where Matt went first. His attire had changed now. He actually looked like a doctor. He wore a white jacket that held his stethoscope when it wasn't hanging around his neck. He carried a small leather case that contained an otoscope for looking in ears and an opthalmoscope for looking in the eyes. He had a supply of tongue blades to use to look in the patient's throat and he carried a *Merck Manual*, the medical student's bible, a synopsis of diagnosis and treatment. His immediate boss was a medical intern, Dr. Bill King. The chief medical resident was Dr. Allan Reynolds.

When a new patient is admitted to the medical service, one of the medical students is assigned to do a history and physical. Most medical students hang around the nurse's stations on the medical floors, reading charts and comparing notes while they wait for their cases. Matt was sitting in a chair at the nurse's station when the head nurse, Miss Amy Jones, hollered over to him.

"Dr. Matt Kendall, you're up next. We have a patient coming up from the ER in CHF."

Matt sat bolt upright in the chair. Incredible! His first patient. He suddenly became excited. "Great!" he exclaimed. "I'm going to see my first patient." But he thought for a minute. What the devil is CHF? He turned to the young man next to him. "Mort, what's CHF?"

"Dummy, CHF is congestive heart failure."

He wondered if he would have time to go to the bathroom and read up on congestive heart failure before the patient arrived on the floor. No, he'd better hang around.

Before he really had time to think, the elevator doors opened and a patient sitting upright on the stretcher was whisked in front of the nurse's station. He was an elderly man, gasping for air, looking quite apprehensive and cyanotic. He was quickly wheeled into a room and put into a bed. Matt moved slowly to the door, shuffling uncertainly, and then he thought, hey, you're his doctor, start acting like one. He turned the corner and strode into the room. When he got a good look at the patient he thought for gosh sakes, getting a history from this patient will be impossible. He can't even breathe, let alone answer questions. He was sitting bolt upright in the bed, wobbling slightly, to and fro.

"Should I give him oxygen?" asked the nurse.

"I guess so."

"What do you mean, I guess so? Should I or shouldn't I?"

"Give the oxygen," he replied. He suddenly realized that he had to be positive in his actions. He was the captain of the ship. "Where's Bill King, the intern?"

"He's probably in the rack sleeping," said the nurse.

"Page him stat, please," he said as the nurse left the room and then came back.

"What do you want me to do?" he asked.

"Why don't you listen to his chest and take his blood pressure," she replied with a sarcastic look.

Matt put his stethoscope on the patient's chest. He didn't hear much except some gurgles. The breath sounds weren't normal. He took the patient's blood pressure. It was 230 systolic over 110 diastolic. He thought he'd better check it again to make sure, and got the same result. "Wow!" he exclaimed.

The patient gave him a dirty look.

"Well, what did you find?" asked the elderly nurse.

"He sounds congested."

"Hurrah!" she said. "You've got a little potential. I can look at him and tell that. Should we run a strip?"

A strip? Should he show his ignorance and ask the nurse what a "strip" was? After all, a strip could mean a lot of different things. He decided that a certain level of ignorance was his privilege and he was quickly learning a whole new verbiage.

"What's a strip?" he asked.

"It's an EKG, an electrocardiogram, dummy," she replied.

"Hmm, that's not a bad idea. The only trouble is I don't know how to read one."

"Well, if you're going to be a doctor, you're going to have to learn. Bill King will look at it. He'll be here shortly."

Matt looked at the patient and he seemed to be getting worse. He was puffing harder and getting bluer.

Bill King entered the room, looking somewhat disheveled, but his eyes were alert.

"Well, Dr. Kendall, what do you think is going on here?" he asked.

"He's congested," replied Matt. "He may have had a heart attack."

"Well, you're half right. He's one of our old patients. Have you looked at his old chart?"

"No. I didn't know he had one."

"You should always look at the old chart, if you have time. He's had an old myocardial infarct. The heart attack damaged his heart muscle. The EKG doesn't show anything new. What else have you noticed?"

"He's got high blood pressure."

"How high?"

"Through the roof. Two-hundred-thirty over one-hundred-ten," he replied.

"Don't editorialize when we're discussing a patient. Now, just tell it how it is. Try to put it all together."

"Well, he's got a bad heart from his old heart attack and the pump can't push as well so he's become congested in his lungs. His high blood pressure doesn't help either."

"Right," said Dr. King. "What are we going to do about it?"

"We have to dry him out some way."

"What do you suggest?"

"I'd probably give him a diuretic," said Matt. "Give him some Mercurhydrin to get him to pass his water and get some of the fluid out of his lungs."

"Good. Anything else?"

"Give him something to make the heart muscle function better."

"He's on digitalis. Any other ideas?"

"Give him oxygen."

"He's on oxygen. What do you hear in his chest?" asked Dr. King.

"A lot of rattles."

"What are they due to?"

"He's got fluid in his lungs."

"Good," said Dr. King. "Are there any medicines that will help the lungs directly?"

"Not that I know of."

"Well, Aminophylline helps. It's a smooth-muscle relaxant. Or you can tap into the chest with a needle and take the fluid out directly. However, he should have a chest x-ray first."

Dr. King spoke to the nurse. "Order a stat portable chest x-ray. And get me a vial of Aminophylline." Matt noticed that the nurse gave no lip to Dr. King. He realized then that just as he earned his wings in the air, he'd have to earn them down here, too.

"There are a few other diagnostic measures that you can do, Dr.

Kendall. You can put rotating tourniquets on the extremities for a short while to reduce the peripheral resistance and increase the venous flow back to the heart. The heart won't have to pump as much blood around."

"Anything else we should do?" asked Matt.

"We can phlebotomize the patient by taking some blood off. That works dramatically sometimes. Can you think of some other things to do?"

"No," replied Matt. He felt he had reached his level of incompetence.

"We might have to put a Foley catheter into his bladder if he has trouble passing his water. Some of these old guys have big prostates and they have trouble peeing. You're going to have to watch him closely, Dr. Kendall. He's pretty sick."

"Yes sir," he replied.

Matt did watch the patient closely, going in and out of his room several times every hour. He was almost as apprehensive as the patient. The patient did have trouble passing his water and needed a Foley catheter. His chest also had a lot of fluid in it. Matt tapped it with a needle and obtained three quarts of fluid. He also took a pint of blood off. A chest x-ray was taken and a large mass was found in the right lung. Cancer cells were present in the lung fluid. The patient slowly went downhill and died five days later.

Matt went to the pathology department and watched the autopsy. It was a real learning experience. The patient had diffuse spread of a lung cancer which had complicated his heart disease. He was a heavy cigarette smoker and had continued to smoke after his heart attack. It was obvious he didn't listen to his doctor.

Matt's first patient died. But oddly, he didn't feel the remorse he thought would accompany the loss. Death, in this case, made its own kind of sense: the man's body was ravaged and could not function.

In the summer, most medical students try to find a job to earn money to help defray medical school costs or to increase their expertise in medicine. Matt was beginning to think his personality fit that of a surgeon. Surgeons see problems and solve them by operating; he liked the intervention, the active role of healer. He also wanted to find out if he had the stomach to stand the sight of bleeding and whether he was capable of handling the intense stress of the operating room.

A summer surgical fellowship for students who had completed their third year was offered at Genesee, an excellent small general hospital in the middle of Rochester. He had spent a six-week rotation there and knew the food was good, the working conditions great, and there was a solid group of attending surgeons.

If he got the job, he knew he would be the scut boy (the lowest man on the totem pole) and menial tasks would befall him. He would learn how to put needles into veins, suture lacerations, insert stomach tubes prior to gallbladder and stomach surgery, and, if he was lucky, hold retractors on some of the big operations. He'd also get to see inside the abdomen of sick patients and watch the various techniques of the surgeons. He'd work a 12-hour shift and have Mondays off because the weekends were busiest in the emergency room. He would also scrub on weekend emergency cases.

Matt soon found out that emergency cases could be very exciting. He also learned that the intern liked to catch up on his sleep. This meant that he would get to do some of the suturing and see patients from midnight to 6 A.M.

Many of the cases seen were the result of family fights or drunken street corner brawls. There was lots of sewing to do. Matt found the drunks were easier to sew up because most of them didn't feel pain. Some DOAs came in by ambulance. Matt saw them all: heart attacks, knife wounds, gunshot victims, motorcycle accidents.

Some of the smaller hospitals had their own ambulances or worked with private ambulance services. Interns and fourth-year medical students rode the ambulances so that care could be upgraded. Most ambulance cases are routine and can be handled with minimal care. Occasionally, an unusual case will be seen and a life-threatening event develops.

Part of an extern's job at the hospital was to ride the ambulance at night, wearing white trousers and white jacket. Matt didn't like the responsibility of having to face unknown problems, even though there was radio contact with the doctors in the hospital emergency room.

On Saturday night the ambulance got a call to go to the site of a carnival that was in town. A man was having convulsions.

That's great, thought Matt. What do you do for convulsions? He remembered you always put a tongue blade in their mouth so they don't injure their tongue. He also remembered the intern telling him to always look like a professional in front of people or at least try to give the impression that he knew what he was doing.

The ambulance crew was told the man was on the ground near the ferris wheel. The ambulance arrived on the scene with its siren blaring and lights flashing. There was a crowd of people standing around in a circle. In the center was a man lying on his back, his arms and legs thrashing.

"Does anyone know this man?" Matt asked.

"He's alone," replied one of the onlookers.

Matt tried to put a tongue blade between the man's teeth as he continued to convulse. There was mucous drooling from his mouth.

God! What do I do now, he wondered? He remembered to look professional so he put his stethoscope over the man's lungs. That didn't tell him anything. He felt foolish. He looked to see if he had a head wound. The man kept kicking violently.

"Let's see if he's got a wallet," said Matt. "We have to find out more about him."

The attendant opened his wallet and looked through it. The patient continued to convulse. Matt remembered that phenobarbitol was sometimes given to epileptics and he thought about administering some. If his diagnosis was wrong he could kill the patient.

"Hey, Doc. He's got a prescription in his wallet for some medication."

Matt recognized the name of the doctor, who was an endocrinologist at the University. He looked at the prescription. He couldn't read the doctor's handwriting.

"Draw up that fifty percent glucose," he said to the attendant, "and hold his arm still. Giving him intravenous sugar won't kill him."

A tourniquet was put on the arm and Matt injected the glucose into the vein. Suddenly the convulsions stopped. The patient regained consciousness and there was a cheer from the crowd.

"Are you a diabetic?" asked Matt.

"Yes. I guess I took too much insulin today."

"Why don't you wear an emergency bracelet?"

"I used to have one but I lost it," he replied.

"Well, we better take you back with us and get your diabetes under control." Matt smiled as he felt beads of sweat course down his face.

He came to enjoy riding the ambulance at night. He got paid and was called "doctor" by the ambulance personnel and nurses. The big problem that went with the job was the unpredictability. There was much hurried reading and frantic flipping through pages of books that gave summaries telling how a doctor should respond to a given situation. Unfortunately, the books never addressed the details.

Finally, Matt drew the Friday night ride in the ambulance, considered the busiest and most dangerous time. At 7:30 they got an emergency call from one of the posh seafood restaurants in town. A man was choking.

Matt didn't like what he heard. He wasn't ready for this one. The ambulance pulled up to the restaurant. He carried his medical bag and the attendants carried the oxygen tank as they ran into the restaurant.

When he got inside a man was lying on the floor, coughing and gasping for air. It looked as though a woman had passed out next to him. There wasn't much light and it was difficult to see his skin color. The attendant put a flashlight on him. The man was frothing at the mouth, trying to get his breath.

"Oxygen," Matt said to the attendant.

He first tried to look in his throat. "What happened?" he hollered to the people in the restaurant.

"He was drinking quite a few martinis and choked on his food," a waiter said.

Probably a piece of steak or fish caught in his throat, thought Matt. The guy didn't look good. He was beginning to check out.

Matt tried to put his finger into the man's mouth and thought he could feel something. He knew he couldn't get it out without adequate light or instruments. The patient was getting weaker and less reactive.

"Do we have a trach set?" he shouted to the attendants.

"Yes we do," replied the ambulance attendant.

"Open the set up."

He remembered talking to the surgical resident about doing a trach to relieve respiratory obstruction and had scrubbed on an elective tracheostomy in the hospital. God! Now he wished he had watched it more closely. He had never done one.

He also remembered the surgical resident asking him, "Have you ever seen a tracheostomy?"

"No," he replied.

"Well, if you have to take care of an airway obstruction you may have to do one. The only advice I'll give you is that if you ever have to do one, make your incision up and down just under the Adam's apple. When you get to the cartilage of the trachea use a heavy scissors or a sharp knife to cut through it. It can be difficult. Once you start doing a trach just keep going until it's done and work as fast as you can and disregard the bleeding."

Well, the moment of truth had arrived. He knew the man lying on the floor in the restaurant was going to die unless he could get air into his windpipe. His body was getting flaccid.

Matt put on sterile gloves.

"Find me a scalpel," he hollered to the attendant. "Shine the flashlight on his neck. Someone get some more lights!"

With his hand shaking, he made an up-and-down incision beneath the Adam's apple. The patient didn't move. He remembered the intern telling him to forget about the blood—if he's dead he won't bleed.

Matt cut deeper. The blood was dark and there wasn't much of it. The patient was still. He didn't react to the knife. He looked dead. Matt put his left forefinger in the wound and felt the cartilaginous windpipe. Make the cut big enough, he remembered. He cut it deeper and longer.

"You got any clamps?" he hollered.

"Here's a Kelly clamp," said the attendant.

Matt put the big clamp in the deep cut and spread it. He tried to cut through the cartilage of the windpipe. Nothing happened. He shoved the knife deeper—hard. He knew he had to make a hole in the windpipe. Suddenly there was a big cough and a bloody mucous plug spat into his face. The patient started to bleed around the wound and air whistled in and out.

"Let's have that trach tube."

The attendant gave him the curved metal tube. The patient started to thrash about.

"Hold him down," he hollered.

It was difficult to see. Matt had a tough time trying to find the opening in the windpipe because of the bleeding. He had to do it. He just had too! He kept holding the Kelly clamp open. He finally spread the clamp as wide as possible and shoved the trach tube gently between the clamp. Luckily, somehow it went into the airway. He quickly tied the string attached to the tube around the back of the man's neck and put the oxygen mask over the opening.

"All right. Let's move. Let's get him to the hospital as quickly as possible. This guy's bleeding like a stuck pig."

They put him in the ambulance and radioed the ER.

"I got a guy coming in with a trach, bleeding heavily," said Matt. "We'll need immediate help on arrival."

When they got the patient to the emergency room, he was taken to the operating room and the chief surgical resident quickly clamped and tied the vessels around the airway. He was given a unit of blood and intravenous antibiotics. An ENT doctor came in and removed a fish bone from his throat. It looked like he had swallowed half the fish.

The ENT guy shook his head. "When these people drink too much their throats become anesthetized. If they don't chew their food properly they try to swallow a chunk of food too big and choke to death. It's usually either steak or fish bones that do the damage. You did a good job, Matt."

"There's got to be a better way to take care of a choking patient," he replied. "I didn't think I had the guts to do what I did."

"I'm sure there will be, in the future," said the ear, nose, and throat doctor.

Matt's fourth year in medical school went by very quickly. He rotated through the medicine, surgery, obstetrics, and pediatric services. His responsibilities had increased in the care of patients, although he was still under controlled supervision—either an intern or resident would have to initial his histories, physicals, and progress notes. He now had more hands-on diagnostic experience in the care of patients and a greater part of the year was taken up in actual patient care. He delivered his first baby on the obstetrical service; took care of patients with acute coronaries; saw young children die from meningitis; participated in the care of major trauma cases in the emergency room. He was the low man on the totem pole so that scut work was assigned to him by his superiors, usually the intern on his service.

All scut work had to be done early in the morning prior to going into the operating room or making bedside rounds with the professors. It was time consuming and considered a pain in the ass by most students because it offered very little to improving diagnostic acumen.

The most important decision that Matt would make in his fourth year was where he would apply for an internship. The best hospitals in the country, such as Mass. General, Johns Hopkins, University of Pennsylvania, University of Michigan, and the University of Pittsburgh have no problem getting top-quality interns. Less attractive hospitals have difficulty filling their rosters. Each student wants to go to the best hospital they qualify for. However, there are a limited number of spaces available. This leads to a disruptive and chaotic mess when a decision has to be made by the hospital and student.

The year that Matt graduated from medical school, a new system was devised for the selection of hospitals and interns—The National Intern Matching Plan. In this plan the student rated the hospitals that he wanted to go to and the hospital rated the students.

The medical students and hospitals were matched by computer on March 15 and the students and hospitals were informed where the student would be taking postgraduate training. Not every student was matched to where he wanted to go, and not every hospital received the students they wanted.

There were two basic types of internships available to choose from: A *straight internship*—all medicine or surgery—or a *rotating internship*—where the intern rotated through different services with an emphasis on medicine or surgery. There were two different types of hospitals to apply to; one was an academic hospital attached to a medical school where full-time professors did most of the teaching, and the other was a general or city hospital where most of the physicians and surgeons were in private practice—the teaching was not as intense but the responsibility was greater.

Most of the large general hospitals or city hospitals were the bastions of training for the student who eventually went into general practice. This type of hospital also attracted students who were not sure what field of medicine they wished to spend the rest of their lives in.

Matt had met and dated Nancy Smith, a beautiful brown-eyed brunette from West Virginia, and was planning to get married at the end of his senior year. His marriage to Nancy would have an influence on which hospital he would apply to.

There were two ways to find out. One was to take a fellowship for a month during the fourth year at a hospital that he might want to go to. This would allow the hospital to meet him and evaluate his skills. It also would allow him to see if he wanted to go there for his training.

The second way was to take a trip during the Christmas vacation to look at the hospitals that he might be interested in and to have an interview.

His medical advisor suggested that he visit five hospitals. The Mayo

Clinic in Rochester, Minnesota; the University of Chicago; Detroit
Receiving Hospital; Bellevue Hospital in New York City; Whitestone
Hospital in New England.

The hospitals were selected so he could get a kaliedoscopic view of
medical school academics and big-city hospital training.

He took a plane to the Mayo Clinic for his first stop. The rest of the
trip would be completed by train.

When the plane landed on the runway in Rochester, Minnesota, he
took a cab and he checked into the Kaylor hotel, which was the only
hotel in town, and was pleasantly surprised that a copy of the next
day's operating schedule was available for visiting surgeons. He visited
St. Mary's Hospital, the largest hospital affiliated with the Mayo
Clinic, and was impressed with the large volume of surgery. The
attending surgeons were doing most of it. He talked to some of the
resident surgical fellows and found out that they did very little surgery
except for opening and closing wounds.

While on a train to Chicago he wrote down his impressions about
the Mayo Clinic. The bottom line was: Outstanding attending staff—
very little actual operating done by the resident staff.

After arriving in the city of Chicago, he went to visit the University
of Chicago. He was impressed by the physical plant, a magnificent
high-rise structure. The university had a reputation for an excellent
medical staff that did outstanding research. When you entered the
lobby of the hospital you were impressed with its opulence. You were
even more impressed when you saw the surgical operating suites with
the latest technical equipment.

One of the associate professors of surgery interviewed Matt and sat
down and had a long chat with him. He asked, "Are you interested in
doing research?" It was the first time that anyone had asked that
question.

"I really don't know. I haven't given it very much thought," Matt
replied.

"Well, if you come here for surgery, you'll have to spend a year or two
doing basic research," said the professor. "It will make you a better
doctor and help your academic career. If you eventually do productive
research, it will allow you to give something back to society."

"I'm not so sure that I want to add two more years to my training.
I've already given up four years of my life."

The professor was taken aback by his reply. He said, "You mean
you've already spent four years in medical school?"

"No. I don't mean that at all! I spent four years of my life as a night torpedo bomber pilot in the Atlantic and Pacific during the war. I'm trying to catch up."

"That's too bad," said the professor. "We have one of the best research laboratories in the country."

That evening, Matt met a medical school classmate of his at the YMCA where he was staying and they decided to go over to the stockyard area and have a steak. Bill Kyte was in Chicago to look over Northwestern University.

"How are you making out in your travels?" he asked.

"I was impressed with Northwestern Hospital in the city," he said. "Although I like the smaller hospital out in the suburbs in Evanston. How about you, Matt? Did you talk to any of the interns or residents at the University of Chicago?"

"I did. They have a pyramid system. You don't get to do much surgery until you get to the senior level or when you're chief. The University of Chicago is quite impressive but I've scratched it off my list."

"Why?"

"If I took a residency in surgery there, it would take me an extra year or two—and I don't have those years to give. They require that you do an extra year or two doing basic surgical research. Where are you heading next?" he asked.

"I'm going to Denver to look at the University of Colorado. How about you?"

"Detroit Receiving Hospital, right in the heart of Detroit—right in the ghetto. I hope I can get in and out of there alive."

"That ought to be an interesting hospital to look at."

"Yeah, it's a big-city hospital with lots of action."

Matt arrived in Detroit late on a Friday afternoon, had a brief interview with an attending surgeon, and was assigned an intern to show him around.

"I'm working in the ER this evening," said the intern. "Why don't you come back after supper? You can see what the hospital is really like. Ask for Margie. I'll tell her you're coming."

Matt got a bite to eat and came back at 7:30.

When he walked into the emergency room, everything seemed to be in disarray. There was a man lying on a stretcher in front of the nurses' station holding his side, moaning. No one seemed to be paying any attention to him.

He looked around for Margie—there were no nurses that could be seen—let alone Margie. A big black woman sat behind the nurses' station desk reading a newspaper—oblivious to whatever was taking place.

Matt got up enough nerve to talk to her. "Where are all the nurses?"

"We just had a code one," said the secretary. "They're all down in room eight. What are you doing around here?"

"I'm a fourth-year medical student. I'm here to see Dr. Scussel, one of the interns."

"He's down there too," she said. "You can go down to room eight and see what's going on, if you like."

Matt walked down to room eight, which looked like a large examining room that had been converted into an operating room. Stretched out on an operating table under a big light was a big black man with a chest wound that was bleeding profusely. Somebody had gotten a tube down his throat and was trying to pump oxygen into him. A nurse was holding a metal retractor against a rib so the surgical resident or intern could try to locate the bleeding.

Matt found out who Margie was in a hurry. "Don't just stand there," she hollered. "Help me pump blood into this guy's IV."

"We're gonna need some chest tubes, Margie," said the surgical resident.

"They're on the table," she said.

He grabbed one and shoved it into the opening in the wound. "Any more visible stab wounds?"

"I can't see any more, Jim."

"How's his pressure?"

"It's back up to 90/60."

"We have to close him up down here."

Matt decided to speak up. "Why don't you take this guy up to the operating room?"

"Cause the operating rooms are filled," said the surgical resident. "We've had a shootout at OK Corral and a couple of other stabbings in the ghetto. Put a pair of gloves on and help us close."

After the wound was closed, the patient was transferred upstairs to the recovery room.

"If he bleeds anymore tonight, we'll crack his chest, when one of those operating rooms opens up," said the surgical resident.

The next day, Matt eventually met the director of the training program. He sat down and talked to him.

"You interested in trauma?" he asked.

"Maybe."

"Well, here's the place to go then. We have trouble keeping up with the amount we get. Any questions you want answered?"

"Yes. How do I know if I have a chance to get an internship here?"

"I think you've got a shot at it."

With that comment, Matt was dismissed.

The next morning he took a train to New York City. His next stop would be Bellevue Hospital, down on the lower east side of New York. After seeing Detroit Receiving, he wondered what Bellevue would be like. When the train pulled into Grand Central Station, he hailed a cab. "Bellevue Hospital, please."

The cab driver turned around, looked him in the eye and said: "What do yah wanna go der fer?"

"I'm thinking about taking some training there as an intern," he replied.

"I wouldn't do it, if I was you," said the cabbie.

When the cab pulled up to the front door of Bellevue, Matt's first impression was not inspiring. It was a drab-looking brick and stone building. He entered a room that needed new rugs and paint. It was a marked contrast to the Mayo Clinic and the University of Chicago—even Detroit Receiving. He walked through some dingy hallways to a small office that had a small sign on the outside—Dr. Louchello, Chief of Surgery. Matt had a brief interview with him and then was taken around the wards by one of the first assistant surgical residents—a Dr. Clifford Ward.

He told Matt that he was an Iowa farmboy who made the mistake of wanting to become a surgeon at Bellevue. Matt was taken aback by that statement. He took a closer look at him. He looked as though he needed a bath and had that glassy-eyed look of chronic fatigue. He was having difficulty keeping his eyes open and yawned frequently.

"Where are you from, Kendall?"

"Connecticut," he replied.

"Why do you want to come to this big, filthy metropolis?"

"I think I may want to be a surgeon."

"If I were you, I'd forget it! You either want to be a surgeon or you don't—thinking's no good! How's your health?"

"Good."

"You married?"

"Gonna be soon."

"Well, if you come here, you might get TB and if you get married—you won't be by the time you finish training."

Matt looked at him with a quizzical stare. "What do you mean by that?"

"You're on your own. You don't get a lot of supervision but you get a lot of responsibility—early! You'll know how and where to cut if you make it—if you don't—they'll throw you out on your ass. Do you want to see one of the surgical wards?"

"Yes."

He took Matt to one of the wards, a large room filled with patients. It looked like they were all deathly sick. There was no privacy. Most of the patients had stomach tubes, IVs, chest tubes, and Foley catheters. Matt noticed there weren't too many nurses.

"Do you want to see our ER?"

"No thanks. I saw enough out in Detroit."

The surgical resident looked at Matt and then said sarcastically, "Well, Kendall, you coming here?"

"I've got to give it a lot of thought," he replied.

The next day, Matt took a train to his last stop—Whitestone Hospital in the middle of Connecticut.

What a contrast to Bellevue and Detroit Receiving! The hospital was sparkling white—almost brand new—about thirteen stories high. The entrance had marble floors. It was almost like a Taj Mahal.

He couldn't believe they called this a city hospital—everything was so new and immaculate. The city hospitals that he had seen were dumps compared to this. The internship they offered was a two-year rotating internship with the second year an emphasis in medicine or surgery.

He met Dr. John Leone, the medical program director, a man with a small mustache who had an exuberant enthusiasm about his training program. He also met Dr. Phillip McBratney, one of the chiefs of surgery, who had trained at Johns Hopkins. He was shown the operating room floor that had 30 operating rooms and met Dr. Jack Cox, the chief resident, who seemed to be well rested and quite relaxed.

When he was standing alone with Dr. Cox, he asked him whether he liked the hospital.

"I think it's a great hospital—good teaching, good supervision, and responsibility. There's only one drawback, they don't pay you and there's a lot of scut work."

"That's true of all good programs, isn't it?"

"That's right," said Jack. "Unless you have someone with big bucks backing you, it's tough to become a surgeon here, unless you want to live in poverty."

When Matt got back to Rochester, he talked to his advisor and then had a long talk with Nancy.

Detroit and Bellevue would be rough for Nancy. The Mayo Clinic or Chicago might be better. It would be a long, drawn-out process before he would get any responsibility in an academic setting. Whitestone would allow him to get an early taste of surgery. If he didn't like surgery, he could become a G.P. It was a beautiful hospital with a well-trained diversified staff and an excellent teaching program. He and Nancy decided that Whitestone Hospital would be his first choice.

4

ON MARCH 15TH, The Match took place. Matt was lucky—he got his first choice. He would be going to Whitestone Hospital. He called Nancy, and told her the good news.

"Oh, Matt, that's great," she said. "Now we can get married."

Nancy had vitality, strength, and intelligence and she believed in Matt. For Matt it was a departure from all he'd known, for Nancy had unshakable faith in his goal to become a doctor. No one, not even his family, had ever endorsed his pursuits unreservedly. For Matt, it was enough. More, in fact, then he could have hoped for.

Their wedding was held in a large church on East Avenue in Rochester. Nancy's family turned out in force. Matt's family and the entire medical school graduating class was in attendance. As the two were showered with rice, they hopped into their car and drove to Williamsburg, Virginia for their honeymoon.

Matt's transition from medical school to internship was not easy. In medical school his first two years were spent studying for hours on end—big, complicated medical books in the library. During the last two years he found out what medicine was all about—taking care of the sick, the maimed, and the hopelessly poor. He saw what trauma and disease could do to the human body and he experienced the frustration of some of his patients dying.

His new lifestyle as an intern had changed more drastically. He was now on call at the hospital every other night and every other weekend—working 120 hours a week without pay. His mental and physical capacities were being tested to their zenith degree.

To help pay the bills, Nancy got a job working on the medical floors at Whitestone Hospital. She was not only a pretty brunette with big brown eyes, she was an intelligent, well-trained nurse. Matt's long working hours as an intern were not an ideal situation conducive to a happy marriage, but they made the most of it when they were together.

Working in a high-stress atmosphere for more than twenty-four hours straight led to the fulfillment of the concept work hard, play hard. Being young and in good health helped. They found a small clean, inexpensive furnished apartment under a third-floor roof. Nancy had to learn to cook, which was not difficult since they had to subsist on simple food such as macaroni and cheese and spaghetti and meatballs. Fortunately, she was able to arrange her schedule so she was off when Matt was off. They were in the minority in the internship group. Most of the interns were single—marriage was frowned upon by the hospital administration. There were only three other married couples in the group of twenty-four interns.

Each year in July there was a welcoming party for the incoming group. It was a splash party given by the chief of radiology at his beautiful spacious home in the suburbs. The grounds were magnificent and the swimming pool was olympic size. A softball game was played, then followed by a dip in the pool. Fine food, beer and wine were plentiful. Many of the pretty young nurses at Whitestone were invited to the party. This allowed for a more intimate evaluation of some of the young nurses' physical attributes.

The chief of radiology had two beautiful daughters who were also invited.

One of the veteran interns knew a good thing when he saw it and ended up spending the evening on a blanket under the moon with the youngest daughter.

Their engagement was announced six weeks later. Bill Carlson, the intern, took a ribbing about that. Suddenly, he went from poverty to high-society status and it wasn't long before he announced that he was going to take a residency in radiology.

However, the Whitestone nurses didn't lose out altogether with the incoming interns. For identification purposes, the interns' pictures were pinned up at the nurses' stations on each floor at the hospital. The young nurses quickly wrote the marriage status underneath each picture. This led to frequent weekend intern-nurse get-acquainted parties where the liquor flowed along with whatever. The funding for the parties came from contributions by the working girls.

Since the young doctors had studied anatomy intensely in medical school, it wasn't too long before they applied their knowledge to their social life. The nurses had also taken courses in the subject. It was not unusual at some of the parties that a more intimate study of each other's anatomy took place.

During the first year, six of the young interns succumbed to the tantalizing characteristics and ravishing beauty of the Whitestone nursing staff and got married.

Nancy and Matt would occasionally have a couple of the single interns and their dates over for dinner on the weekends. They became close friends with two of the interns. Nick was an intern who was secretly married to a student nurse from Boston. If the nursing school found out she was married, she would be dropped from the training program. When Matt and Nancy were working on a weekend, the couple would occasionally use their apartment.

The other was John Ball, a single veteran who was a sergeant in the Air Force during the war. He was dating a very pretty student nurse. John and Matt needled each other quite often about their war flying experiences. John had flown over the mountains in India in DC-3s and was a great storyteller. After quite a few drinks at one of the interns' parties, he told a terrific story about when his plane was shot down.

Because John was the sergeant in charge of the men doing the manual tasks in the back of the plane, it was his duty to jump out last if the plane got shot up and they had to bail out. Well, it happened. Six enemy planes were waiting for them on one of their missions over the Himalaya mountains and both of their engines were shot up and destroyed.

The plane was at seventeen thousand feet. "We were told by the pilot to bail out," said John. He was the last one to jump as the plane descended vertically in a dive. Part of the tail assembly hit him on the side of his head and knocked him unconscious before he could pull the rip cord on his parachute. He came to as he dropped down from the sky and suddenly realized that he was in a free fall and his chute wasn't open. He pulled the rip cord at 1,000 feet and landed in a clump of trees tangled in his parachute. He was hanging from his parachute when a tribe of Indian natives arrived and put a primitive ladder up to his parachute to release him. When he got to the ground, the natives got down on their knees and bowed their heads. They thought he was a god descending from the heavens. John didn't understand their language and they didn't understand his but he was glad that he wasn't killed by their spears. He was brought to the tribal chief and placed on an elevated throne in the center of the village and the natives presented him with all sorts of gifts. "That was just the beginning of my problems," said John. The group of interns intently leaned forward and listened. "That evening I was given my own primitive hut to stay in.

"The real shocker came when the tribal chief brought his daughter to my hut and offered her as an evening companion. How can you refuse that," asked John, "without offending the chief?"

"What was she like?" asked one of the interns.

"She was the most beautiful woman I had ever seen," he replied, "dark skinned and gorgeous."

"How did you make out?" asked the group.

"It was a disaster," he replied. "The problem was, she really was underfed. She was five feet tall and weighed over 200 pounds and the ugliest thing I had ever seen."

"What did you do?" they all asked in unison.

"I couldn't refuse," replied John. "I was stuck with a *big* problem. She had been instructed by her father what to do and to acquiesce to the god's wishes.

"I spent most of the evening trying to fend off that baby buffalo.

"I finally decided to stick my finger down my throat to try to vomit, but it didn't work.

"She thought it was some ritual to do before you have sex. After she completely disrobed she kept sticking her finger down her throat."

"Tell us the truth, John," said one of the interns. "What did you do?"

"I made believe I was really sick. I moaned and groaned, writhing on the floor. The baby buffalo got the message. She got dressed and left the hut."

"You were lucky on that one," commented Bill Hill.

"Not really," replied John. "She returned with the tribal medicine man who had the most grotesque mask over his face. That was to drive away the evil spirits that were causing my illness," said John. "He also had some kind of root medicine he wanted me to swallow."

"Did you drink it?" asked the interns.

"Are you kidding? Some of those root medicines have poison in them.

"The medicine man insisted I drink it. I still refused. I pointed to the chief's daughter to drink it and she did."

"What happened?"

"Just what I thought would happen. She got sick and vomited all over my hut. That took care of her for the first night."

"So, what happened?"

"She came back the next night with a new medicine man with a new mask on his face."

"You gotta be kidding."

"So, finish your story," said the interns.

"I rubbed noses with her and patted her bottom and that was the end of that."

"Yeah. I'll bet," they all said in unison.

Matt's first six-week rotation at Whitestone Hospital was on the general surgical service. He did histories and physicals on patients, started intravenous fluids, ordered medications, and scrubbed on surgical cases when an assistant was needed. Usually that meant holding metal retractors against the abdominal wall and pulling so that the surgeon could see and work better within the depths of the abdomen. The chief resident surgeon would stand opposite the operating attending surgeon and help clamp bleeders, tie vessels, and cut sutures.

Occasionally the attending surgeon would ask questions about the case and Matt would attempt to give a correct answer.

Gallbladders are particularly hard to hold retractors for since the gallbladder is tucked under the surface of the liver. If it's acutely inflamed, everything is stuck together and the surgeon often would holler to pull harder. Matt was quite muscular so he was usually able to leverage enough force to accommodate whoever was operating.

"I think you have a potential to be a good surgeon," said one of the senior surgeons.

Matt looked him in the eye not sure how to respond and then blurted out, "How on earth can you tell that?"

"Because you hold the retractors well," he said. "That means you can stand frustration. It means you'll probably persist in what you're doing. If you can't hold retractors well you'll never be a good surgeon."

Matt thought about that. Was the surgeon just trying to get him to pull harder so it would be easier for him to do his surgery, or did he really mean it? Some surgeons are con artists, he mused.

The next week he was assigned to scrub on a case with the chief of surgery. In the scrub room the chief made some general remarks about surgeons. "Not only do you have to know cognitive skills, you have to know how to use your hands properly." He pointed to the hallway where a young maintenance man was pushing a broom around. "See that man out there? I can teach him how to tie knots better than you'll ever know. However, I don't believe I can teach him *when* to cut, *where* to cut, and *where* to tie knots. A good surgeon has to know how to think on his feet. You're all alone with the patient's life in your hands. There's no library you can use for a reference to describe what you've found and how to treat it when you're operating. Harry Truman once said, 'The buck stops here.' That also applies to a surgeon. Dr. Kendall, are you going to be a medical prognosticator and contemplate your navel, or a thinking surgeon?"

Matt thought for a minute. That was a most unusual question. It was also an intimidating question. He didn't quite know how to answer. "I don't know, sir," he replied.

"Well, we'll soon find out your preference on our service."

Matt got along well with the chief of surgery and eventually assisted him on several cases. He got to tie some knots and to put a few stitches in and by the time he finished his six weeks on the general surgical service he became adept at clamping bleeders, cutting sutures, and learning about sterile technique.

His second rotation was on the urology service. The chief's name was Dr. William Stronghart. He was a tough disciplinarian, and known to be rough on the interns and first-year residents. His voice was like a bullhorn that made the shutters rattle.

Most of the residents called the urology service the plumbing service because the doctors primarily dealt with the water works. The kidneys, ureters, and bladder are vital to a healthy existence because all liquid waste products are excreted through these organs.

One morning, Matt looked at the OR schedule and saw that he would be assisting Dr. Stronghart on a suprapubic resection of the prostate. This would be the biggest case he had scrubbed on alone and he would be scrubbing with the chief of the service. He was apprehensive and he didn't like it.

The patient was a 78-year-old man who had had prostatic obstruction previously on numerous occasions and had BPH (benign prostatic hypertrophy). He also had chronic heart disease and was a smoker. Because of his past history, the anesthesiologist announced the patient couldn't be put to sleep for the operation. He would be given a spinal, which meant he would be awake during the procedure.

Matt decided to be early for the case so he could read the chart and be prepared for any questions Dr. Stronghart might throw at him. He had done the history and physical and a rectal exam so he could feel the prostate gland. It was a large one!

Dr. Stronghart came into the scrub room where Matt was doing his ten-minute scrub prior to surgery.

"Well, Sonny," said Dr. Stronghart. "Have you seen or done any of these cases before?"

"No, sir. This is my first," he replied.

Stronghart looked at him over his glasses—it was a stern, measured gaze. "Have you read up on the anatomy?"

"Yes, sir."

"Did you order any blood for this operation?"

"Yes, sir, two units, sir. Will that be enough?"

"I should hope so," replied Dr. Stronghart. "Did Dr. Russo, the cardiologist, see him in consultation?"

"Yes, sir. There's a long note on the chart."

"That's not good!" said Dr. Stronghart. "When there's a long note on the chart it either means the patient has a serious cardiac problem or the heart specialist doesn't know what's wrong with him. What did he say about his cardiac status?"

"Well, he has a first-degree heart block that he's had for a long time. He's probably had a coronary in the past because of the changes in his electrocardiogram. He cleared him for surgery."

"What was on the bottom line?"

"He said to try and avoid any serious blood loss if you can."

Stronghart shook his head. "Wonderful," he said.

After doing a ten-minute scrub, Dr. Stronghart and Dr. Kendall walked into the operating room with their arms held high and put on their gowns and gloves. The patient was draped with sterile sheets after the abdomen had been scrubbed with antiseptic solution. The spinal had been done and the anesthesiologist had checked with a pin on the skin to see if the sensory and motor nerves had been knocked out in the lower abdomen.

Matt placed himself opposite Dr. Stronghart and the operating scrub nurse faced him. That was odd, he thought. Usually the scrub nurse is opposite the operating surgeon. Dr. Stronghart raised his forefinger indicating he wanted the knife and pointed to Matt.

The nurse handed the scalpel to Matt. He handed it back to her. Dr. Stronghart took his finger and pointed to the lower abdomen, swinging his finger in a vertical manner as to where the incision was to be made. Again, the nurse handed Matt the scalpel. Again, he gave it back. Stronghart looked at Matt with eyes that could crack granite.

Miss Ross, the scrub nurse, handed the knife back to Matt. He placed the knife just over the pubic bone in the midline of the lower abdomen. Just as he did so, Dr. Stronghart's big right paw covered the top of Matt's hand and he pulled down and guided Matt's hands on the sharp knife all the way through the tissues of the abdomen. The skin split and slid apart and the knife almost nicked the small bowel. There was brisk bright red bleeding all over the place as Dr. Stronghart clamped the blood vessels with Mosquito and Kelly clamps.

"That's how you do it," he bellowed. "Let's tie these up." Silk suture material was handed to Matt. He placed the silk around the clamp held by Stronghart and felt as though he was all thumbs. All that practice tying string around the bed posts was helpful, but it was obvious that he needed more practice on living tissue.

"There are about ninety different types of surgical knots you're going to have to learn, Sonny. You'll have to do two-handed, one-handed, and one-finger ties if you want to be a good surgeon. You'll have to be able to tie a blood vessel automatically, like a machine, even if you can't see the point of the clamp to tie around."

After cutting through the abdominal wall, Matt's incision came down directly over the bladder, which was distended with urine like a big balloon from the chronic obstruction.

Dr. Stronghart grabbed the bladder with two Babcock clamps to lift it up and then, taking heavy scissors, he cut into the bladder. There was more brisk bleeding. He sucked out the urine and blood with a metal-tipped sucker. He then placed two ureteral catheters in the ureters that ran from the kidney, and made an incision around the capsule of the prostate at the base of the bladder, which Matt couldn't see. He then stuck his big, gloved forefinger in the opening and shelled out the large prostate. It took him just a few minutes. The bleeding became more active.

"Prostate surgery is like peeling an orange," said Stronghart.

God, he's rough, thought Matt. How the hell's he going to stop the bleeding? Stronghart grabbed a big metal sucker to suck the blood out and then he cauterized the diffuse bleeding points.

He spoke gruffly to Matt, "Keep sucking this blood out. You better give him another unit of blood," he told the anesthesiologist.

Dr. Stronghart reached under the drapes, and tugged on the Foley catheter to create pressure on the bleeding surface around the prostate. The bleeding subsided with the pressure and cauterization and the placing of suture ligatures. When the bleeding stopped the bladder was closed with a whipstitch of catgut and the abdomen rapidly closed.

"Well, Sonny, now you've seen a suprapubic prostate operation. What do you think of it? Do you think you might want to be a urologist?"

Matt wanted to say it was perhaps the single most disgusting thing he'd seen, but thought better of it. "Well, it certainly is an interesting operation," he responded—and wanted to add—quite bloody!

"Are you on call tonight?"

"Yes, Dr. Stronghart."

"Keep a good eye on him and give him more blood if he needs it."

"Yes, sir," replied Matt. "I sure will."

One of the major strengths of the Whitestone Hospital was its size. It allowed for a diversity of patients.

Matt's first two services were surgical—general surgery and urology—which he enjoyed, and he was giving general surgery a lot of thought as a possible future.

His third rotation was the medical service. He was told by his fellow interns that he'd be getting more sleep because he wouldn't have to get up as early. Part of the rotation on medicine was to spend two weeks in neurology.

During the second weekend of the rotation while he was covering the neurology service, five consecutive patients were admitted with cerebral vascular accidents—strokes of all types. In two cases, it was impossible to get histories. They were elderly men who were rushed to the emergency room by ambulance. Both had fallen and hit their heads and had lacerations and blood over their scalps. They were unable to speak, and no one was with them. In one case, there was no identification because someone had lifted the man's wallet. Another had respiratory difficulty and it was impossible to determine if he had a subarachnoid hemorrhage irritating his respiratory center in the brain. The surgical resident had to be called to do a tracheotomy and respiratory support was given with an oxygen machine.

Sometimes a massive thrombus (clot on the wall of the vessel) or an embolis (clot that travels from the lungs or other sites) obstructs a major blood vessel to the brain and severe irreversible brain damage occurs because nutrients and oxygen, carried by the blood and its elements, cannot reach the brain cells to feed them and keep them alive. In some cases, decompression or burr holes through the bones in the head are used to relieve the increasing pressure caused by the swelling of the brain. It doesn't always work, however.

After staying up all night, doing spinal taps, looking for blood in the spinal column and performing other tests, Matt came home on Monday night and told Nancy that he wasn't going to be an internist or G.P. He was frustrated and felt he had not accomplished anything worthwhile the entire weekend.

"I couldn't help those people. They were gone," he said. "When someone's brain dead, they might as well be shot. They can't see, can't talk, can't communicate, can't walk. It's a godawful mess. Life is not worth continuing in that situation. It's a blessing, as you age, if you maintain your wits and intellect. It's a disaster if you can't."

"Don't make any hasty decisions," replied Nancy.

"I have to commit myself for next year's residency within the next three months," he replied, "or look for a job in general practice."

"Your next rotation is six weeks in neurosurgery, isn't it?"

"Yes."

"Why don't you wait and see what happens on that service?"

"You're right, I will. I'm not looking forward to this rotation. I understand that the chief of neurosurgery is a wild man. The residents and nurses call him Wild Bill Sheridan. He's always on an ego trip—thinks he's God. He yells at the interns and residents on the service constantly. I've been told that most neurosurgeons have a variety of mental problems—and internophobia is one of them."

"Well, don't pass judgment on the neurosurgical department until you've been exposed to it."

During the next three weeks, as he worked on the neurosurgical service, he determined there were three types of patients. *Spinal disk problems* occur when the washer-like disks between the vertebrae compress the nerves coming out of the spine and cause nerve damage down the extremities. These patients usually have severe back or leg pain, and once the ruptured disk is removed, they're like a new person.

Trauma is another major part of the specialty. Automobile and motorcycle accident victims often arrive in the ER with severe head injuries. Many of the cases Matt dealt with were fractured skulls with swelling of the brain that often needed decompression. Frequently there was bleeding within the enclosed skull, which increased the intracranial pressure, causing compression against the brain tissue. Some medications helped but it was usually a wait-and-see situation.

Brain tumors are the most unfortunate cases. If they are malignant, the patient is in for a tough time. Some of the symptoms are subtle—double vision, for example. One of the first signs of a brain tumor is pressure within the skull, sometimes causing persistent headaches, or pressure against the optic nerve, causing changes in the field of vision.

In order to remove a malignant brain tumor, you have to open the skull and surgically remove the tumor. This means you have to cut through normal nerve pathways that can be permanently damaged by invasive surgery. The brain is the human computer center. Most primary brain tumors do not spread to other parts of the body as other malignant tumors do. Malignant tumors from other organs can spread to the brain, however. Lung cancer and breast cancer often do this in the terminal stages of the disease.

Occasionally, some surface tumors of the brain were removed using local anesthesia. After being on the service for three weeks, Matt was assigned to assist the chief of neurosurgery, Wild Bill Sheridan, on a small surface brain tumor that was being removed under local anesthesia.

The brain has its network of blood vessels in a soft, spongy, white substance and it's difficult for the neurosurgeon to control bleeding while operating. You can't go into the skull and tie sutures in the middle of the brain like you do in general surgery—the tie would slice right through the soft brain substance, destroying the tissue.

The patient usually sits up in an operating room chair and his head is shaved. The area around the skull is then injected with a local anesthetic. Drapes are placed around the field of surgery to keep it sterile and a small window is made in the skull with electrical saws. On this particular occasion, the patient was wide awake because the surgeon wanted to see if any motor nerve routes might be damaged as he cut across the tissue.

As they were working, Wild Bill continued to harrass and cajole his chief resident. "You're not putting those patties over the bleeders properly. Watch what you're doing. We're dealing with a man's brain here! For God's sake, help me," he kept hollering. "I can't work properly unless you help me. I'm not a miracle man. I'm not God. Where the hell did you train?"

Matt continued to watch in amazement as the chief neurosurgeon lambasted his chief resident. He concluded that Wild Bill had missed his calling and would have made a great actor—or maybe a hog caller at a rodeo.

The problem facing the neurosurgical team was a serious one. They were having trouble controlling the bleeding, and everyone in the operating room could feel the tension.

Wild Bill was using a fine, pointed needle, and the coagulation device was not stopping the bleeding. He tried using a long, sharp, pointed pick-up to compress the bleeding vessel. The instrument wasn't working properly so he threw it against the wall. He began screaming at the chief resident again. "Help me, doctor. For God's sakes help me! Can't you see the trouble we've got! Help me! Do you want this patient to bleed to death?"

Suddenly there was a movement of the man's head under the drapes. The bleeding increased. He moved his head from under the drapes and spoke up in a loud voice and pleaded, "For God's sake, help the doctor, I don't want to die."

Matt placed a sterile gauze over the open wound in the skull to act as pressure as the others gently positioned the patient back in the chair. When he removed the gauze, the bleeding had almost stopped. The tension ended just as quickly as it had started. The small tumor was removed, the wound was closed, and the operation was a success.

The following week, an incident occurred that hit close to home. Matt's 80-year-old father, who was in the construction business, was building a home in a wealthy suburban area. He was working alone in the upstairs area of the house when he fell two stories and hit his head against the concrete foundation in the basement. He was knocked unconscious, and when he finally came to, he got to his feet, drove his car home, went to his bedroom, and pulled the covers down on his bed.

He had motor nerve function, but he couldn't talk. Fortunately, his daughter was home and called a G.P. to see him. The G.P. called Matt at the hospital. Because the 80-year-old man was aphasic, he was unable to say what had happened to him.

"Matt, it looks like your father has had a stroke. Who do you want to see him?" he asked. "Do you know any of the neurologists?"

"Yes, I do, but shouldn't we have a neurosurgeon see him first?"

"That's all right with me. He's your father. He'll be coming by ambulance to the emergency room. I think it's a medical problem."

"Have Dr. Whitehead take a look at him. He's young but he's a good neurosurgeon."

Matt was in the emergency room when his father arrived. Dr. Whitehead and one of the neurosurgical residents took him aside for a consultation: his father was unconscious and looked to be in pretty bad shape.

"We'll have to do some skull x-rays on him and a spinal tap," said Dr. Whitehead. "I'll call you if we find anything."

As Matt left the ER he looked at his father, unconscious and prone. It was the first time he'd seen him vulnerable, and Matt found himself vindictively regretting that the old man wasn't awake to see, for once, that he needed his son.

As Matt's stare bored into his father's face, he saw a tiny bead of saliva course down his cheek, like a child, and he was ashamed at his anger. In this emotional flux of rage and pity, he returned to the operating room to scrub on another surgical case.

Two hours later he got a call from Dr. Whitehead. "Your father hasn't had a stroke," he said. "He's got a ten-inch fracture at the base of his skull. We're going to take him to the operating room and drill some holes in his skull to decompress the swelling."

Later that night, Matt saw his father. His eyes were open, and he looked alert, but he couldn't talk. The next day he slipped back into a coma. Later that afternoon Dr. Whitehead called Matt again.

"Your father's not doing well. I'd like to do a pneumoencephalogram on him. It's a risky procedure and I'll need your permission."

"Just what is a pneumoencephalogram, anyway?" Matt asked.

"We put air into the ventricles of the brain to see if there's any blood clots in them or displacement. If there is, we suck out the blood that may be compressing the brain substance."

Matt found the decision surprisingly easy, for he knew his father's contempt for weakness and indecision.

"You've got my permission. He's no good the way he is now. He's better off dead."

"I'll call you after we finish operating."

Sure enough, Matt's father had blood filling the left lateral ventricle of his brain and when the blood was removed, he woke up.

The next day, he was fully alert and wanted to get out of bed.

"They don't want you to get out of bed for a couple of days, Dad," said Matt.

"I'm perfectly all right. I can get out of bed."

"Don't prove it. Not until I say so." His father acquiesced, and a moment of understanding, briefly, passed between the two.

He finally became fully ambulatory and started to walk around the neurosurgical ward. He was getting better rapidly. One day, when Matt came into see him, his father was quite agitated.

"Son, I thought you were a good doctor. You've got me on the wrong ward."

"What do you mean?"

"Well, I walked all around this ward today, trying to talk to all the patients. They all have hearing problems. I'd talk to them and none of them would talk back to me. I don't have any hearing problems!"

Matt smiled. When his dad regained consciousness, his own hearing problem was resolved. Most of the patients lying around on the wards had strokes or major brain operations and couldn't speak.

"Dad, most of these patients have had strokes or major brain operations."

"Well, there's nothing wrong with my brain."

Matt sighed. "Of course, but that's a matter of opinion, Dad."

"You little smart aleck. If you were a little younger, I'd spank your behind." With that remark, the old man actually cracked a smile.

After completing the rotation on the neurosurgical service, Matt was assigned back to the general surgical service.

There were two separate surgical services—north and south—and there were two separate chiefs of surgery. On one service Dr. Wallace Stanley was the chief. He had trained at Barnes Hospital in St. Louis and was qualified in general and thoracic surgery. His thoracic surgery training was under Dr. Evarts Graham, who did the first successful lung resection in the United States.

The other surgical chief was Dr. Phillip McBratney, an excellent general surgeon who had trained at Johns Hopkins. Each of the two services had a chief resident surgeon and there were eight assistant surgical residents at different levels of training.

An operating schedule was made up the night before for the following day's surgery and the residents and rotating interns were assigned to specific surgical cases. The interns knew nothing about the capabilities of the attending surgeons they would be working with, so they would ask their fellow interns what to expect. Comments ran the range from terrific to horrifying.

Matt was assigned to assist Dr. Banyon in surgery. He was an elderly surgeon who specialized in vein ligations and strippings. Many times these operations were done on obese women with ugly, dilated veins who wanted their legs to look better. Usually a major branch of the veins (saphenous) was tied off in the upper medial thigh area. A small incision would be made in the lower leg and a metal vein stripper would be passed around the vein and the vein pulled out and stripped out of the leg. Sometimes multiple incisions had to be made because the vein wouldn't come out in one piece. It was often a messy job.

John Ball, Matt's friend, was on the surgical service with him and they often compared notes about upcoming operations.

"Hey, John. What's the book on Dr. Banyon?"

"He's a good real estate man," said John.

"That's not what I'm asking."

"I know. But you better know about it. He owns a tract of land down by the ocean that he's developing and he goes there every weekend. Once he leaves the hospital, he's hard to find."

"Thanks, but what I really want to know is what kind of a surgeon he is."

"He's old fashioned."

"In what way?"

"Well, his cases tend to be bloody, so you'd better order some extra blood before he asks for a scalpel."

"How do you lose a lot of blood on an easy case like a vein ligation and stripping?"

"You'll see. But take my advice and order more than you think you need."

"I'm helping him do bilateral vein ligations tomorrow."

"You got a problem," replied John. "I used to order two pints of blood for one leg, but I only helped him when he did one side. You'd better order double."

Matt took John's advice and ordered four units of blood for the case.

The next day Matt went into the operating room after scrubbing and an assistant held each leg up as he painted them from groin to toe with an antiseptic solution.

Dr. Banyon came in after the patient was asleep and asked, "What's your name, young man?"

"Dr. Matt Kendall."

"Well, Dr. Kendall, if you watch me real close, I'll let you do part of this operation. Maybe even the other leg."

Oh, joy, thought Matt.

Dr. Banyon made an incision in the thigh, tied off the saphenous vein and introduced the metal stripper under the skin and down the medial aspect of the thigh. He made another incision over the end of the stripper and tugged real hard. The vein broke off. He kept making multiple incisions and putting a Kelly clamp in the incision and tearing the vein out. It usually came out in pieces.

The right leg looked like a shrapnel wound or chewed up hamburg. Every time Matt would try to clamp the bleeders Dr. Banyon would say, "Leave them alone. They'll stop. They're only veins."

After completing what Dr. Banyon called a vein ligation and stripping on one leg, he turned to Matt. "Would you like to do the opposite leg?"

"Yes," he replied. He felt anything would be better than what he had just seen.

Dr. Banyon gave the knife to Matt. He delicately incised the left groin and dissected out the saphenous vein and doubly tied it. He then put the metal stripper in and slowly worked it down the thigh, making small incisions and removing the veins. It was a much less messy job but not as professional as Matt wanted it to be.

When they completed the operation, both legs were wrapped in soft gauze padding and ace bandages were taped in place. That evening Matt had to give the patient two units of blood due to blood pooling in the legs because of a big drop in the hematocrit and a drop in blood pressure.

Three weeks later, Matt saw the lady in the hallway of the hospital. He stopped to talk with her. She was using crutches.

"How are you doing, Mrs. Johnson?" he asked.

"OK, except for my right leg. It's a good thing I have a good left leg.

My right leg is still swollen and painful. Dr. Banyon has me on anti-coagulants because of a phlebitis."

"Well, good luck to you," he replied as he walked on and smiled. He had done the left leg.

The next day, Matt looked at the OR schedule and was assigned to hold retractors on a chest case. It was a pneumonectomy for cancer—a lung was to be removed. The operation went very well and the lung was neatly removed and the air tubes (bronchi) to the lungs were sewn up. Just as they started to close the chest wound, a nurse burst into the operating room. "Dr. Starr, come quick! We have a cardiac arrest on a GYN patient down the hall."

Dr. David Starr, the chest surgeon, looked up from his glasses and blurted, "Where? Where?"

"Room six," shouted the nurse.

"Close the chest wound for me, fellows," said the doctor as he ran out of the room and down the hall to room six.

When he got into room six he saw that the anesthesiologist had put a tube through the mouth into the lungs, but the patient was not breathing. She looked blue and was not responding. There was no pulse, heartbeat, or blood pressure. Dr. Starr grabbed a scalpel and made a big incision in the chest. His hand was inside the chest within two minutes and he squeezed the heart in the palm of his hand. Suddenly, the heart began to beat.

The next day Matt heard what had happened.

The chief of gynecology was getting ready to do a D&C (dilatation and curettage) on a 28-year-old who had irregular vaginal bleeding. An intravenous was in place in her arm and the anesthesiologist was putting the patient to sleep. The gynecologist was prepping the vaginal area with an antiseptic solution in preparation for dilating the opening of the cervix to scrape it out. Suddenly, the anesthesiologist said, "I'm not getting a heartbeat."

The gynecologist panicked and screamed at the circulating nurse to get a chest surgeon immediately. The circulating nurse ran out of the room, down the operating room floor to Dr. Starr. He ran back with the nurse and opened the chest with a knife and started massaging the heart. The patient was zapped with electric shock and the heart rate was restored. Unfortunately, when the heart stopped, no oxygen went to the brain and the brain cells were permanently damaged. Her bodily functions returned to normal, but she was unable to respond mentally. This was the first brain-dead patient Matt had ever seen. Her kidney status deteriorated for a while but eventually returned to normal. But she never spoke or recognized anyone again. Her body was in excellent condition but she was gone, lost to the world.

The case was presented to the surgical morbidity and mortality conference and there was an intense inquiry into the management of the case. First the anesthesiologist was questioned about the sodium pentothal and other medications he had used to put her to sleep. Had he given her too much? What precipitated the arrest and caused the heart to stop? Was the medication given too rapidly? Was her airway obstructed? Why wasn't an endotracheal tube put in? In this case, an endotracheal tube was not put down and her breathing was being maintained with a mask. When the arrest occurred, the tube was put down but with some difficulty and delay.

The cardiac arrest occurred as the gynecologist was prepping the cervix. Was she being stimulated in such a manner to cause the heart to fibrillate or have an irregular rhythm? Did the patient go into laryngeal spasm and obstruct her airway? EKG monitors were not in place on this patient because she was assumed to be in excellent health since she was 28 years old.

At the morbidity and mortality conference the chief of surgery spoke up. "This should never happen again! Monitors should be put on all patients prior to surgery, regardless of their age and health. That's now the rule!"

Once the heart stopped, it was obvious the case had been mismanaged. The gynecologist should have opened the chest himself without delay, since adequate oxygen must be circulated to the tissues—particularly the brain. If the tissues do not get oxygen for four to six minutes, permanent brain damage can occur.

5

EACH YEAR, members of the house staff elected officers to represent them in dealing with the attending staff. In his second year, Matt was elected president of the house staff. It was an honorary position, but occasionally meetings to arbitrate a point of dispute between the house staff and the attending staff took place. One of the basic problems was finances.

The interns and residents felt they should be paid something for their services and weren't afraid to make this known. Many times they were scut boys, doing menial tasks without any educational benefits for their services.

Not getting paid for this work was hard to take because the hospital charged for these services. There had to be a better way and the house staff talked about forming a union. Some considered going on strike. They felt a small stipend would help improve their motivation. Eating hospital food was no bargain. There was a limit to the number of relatives who could be brought in for a meal on the holidays; this was a bitter pill for the young doctors. You could bring your wife and/or children for the meal but if you were unmarried you weren't allowed to bring your girlfriend. The bachelor interns were particularly disturbed by this and attempted to change the rules. They'd arrive at the cashier saying, "This is Margie, my new wife," or "this is Sally, my wife." It didn't work. You had to pay cash up front and you would be refunded if you showed a copy of the marriage certificate to the Staff Office.

The biggest holiday event of the year was Thanksgiving. The dining room displayed the traditional Thanksgiving Day feast. It was arranged on a table at the beginning of the cafeteria line. A fully cooked, large turkey with all its trimmings would be displayed with all the condiments and garnishes placed around it. Bottles of champagne and wine were in a basket next to the turkey, along with all sorts of cheeses and crackers and fancy hors d'oeuvres. There was enough there to make your mouth water.

Dr. Johnson, one of the bachelors, suggested to the group of interns that the turkey, with all its fixings, was ready for the taking, and why didn't they just expropriate it, since they all had to work on Thanksgiving Day.

"How do you plan to pull that off?" asked MacDonald, one of the interns.

"It's going to be difficult, but it can be done. Everyone has to be sworn to secrecy because if one guy squeals, we'll all point the finger at him."

"Where are we going to put the turkey?"

"Down the hatch," said Johnson, "Destroy the evidence."

"Sounds like a great idea."

"Let's go over our method of attack."

Six of the interns went over to the barracks and decided on the master plan. There was an elevator that stopped right next to the front of the cafeteria. That would be their exit. A stretcher, complete with sheets and blankets, was obtained from the operating room.

Two interns would man the stretcher and the elevator. They would use the stop button to keep the elevator on the floor next to the turkey. They put false mustaches and dark glasses on and didn't wear their uniforms. Two of the interns went through the line and filled their trays and when they got to the cash register where the head dietician was sitting, they dropped their trays and started a fight. While this was going on, the other interns in the line next to the turkey quickly put the display turkey, champagne, fruit basket, and all the fixings into laundry bags. The elevator doors were opened. The laundry bags were placed on the stretcher and covered with sheets to look like a body and they quickly descended toward the basement.

Unfortunately, the cafeteria was on the second floor and someone had pushed the elevator button on the first floor. A lady was standing there when the doors opened.

"Oh," she gasped, when she saw the sheets over the disguised head and body and the two men who looked like morticians. "I'll take the next elevator."

"That would be wise," said one of the disguised interns.

When they got to the basement, the stretcher was taken to the loading platform, where a girlfriend of one of the interns was waiting with her car. Mud had been thrown over the back license plate. The goodies were taken to her apartment and unloaded, and the turkey was inhaled with French champagne and wine and almost three hours went by before the dieticians realized what happened.

The broken glassware had to be swept up from the floor around the cash register. The two interns who had created the scene were allowed to go back through the line to get refills.

That night, all hell broke loose at the hospital. The head dietician was in a sweat. The president of the attending staff was called in and he interrogated all the interns who were on call. Everyone denied any part in the "turkey caper."

Matt, who was off duty, got a call at home, since he was president of the house staff.

"Dr. Kendall, do you know anything about the theft of the turkey that was on display in the cafeteria?"

"No sir, Dr. Maxwell," he replied. "It's news to me. When did this happen?"

"I'll tell you about it tomorrow," said Dr. Maxwell. "I just wanted to know if you knew anything about it."

"No. I have no idea what you're talking about, sir."

The executive committee of the attending staff was called together and informed about the theft.

One of the chiefs of surgery pounded on the table with his fists and hollered, "Fire them all! They can't be allowed to think they can intimidate us! They're robbers!"

"Who do you suggest we get to replace them?" asked Dr. Maxwell. "Do you want to give intravenous feedings, midnight medicine orders, and do admitting physicals for the next two years?"

"Those scoundrels have to be found and punished," replied the chief of surgery."

"How do you suggest we find them?" asked Dr. Maxwell.

"Call in the Pinkerton detectives and interrogate the interns—all of them separately. There's got to be a weak sister in there somewhere."

"Why don't we start with the president of the house staff council, Dr. Kendall? He's a war veteran and a leader. He'll understand the need for discipline. I'll ask him to meet with us after he gets finished in surgery."

Matt did not like the prospect of meeting with the executive committee—he felt all hell would break loose. The senior medical and surgical officers of the executive committee were seated around the boardroom table. Dr. Maxwell did most of the talking.

"Dr. Kendall, a robbery occurred on Thanksgiving Day. It was quite childish and disgraceful! The display turkey, with all its trimmings, was stolen from the cafeteria. We have reliable information that some of our interns were involved. If you tell us who the participants were, who took part in this robbery, and write a letter apologizing to the attending staff about what happened, the whole matter will be dropped and all will be forgiven. If you don't, this episode will follow you around for the rest of your life and could influence your career."

Matt gave it some thought before he answered. He looked at each doctor straight in the eye.

"First of all, I didn't rob anything. I had the day off! And while I respect all of you, I would not tell you who the culprits were, even if I knew. None of us are paid a living wage. There's quite a bit of unrest in the house staff. This should be a message to you all. I have to live with these men for the rest of the year and the rest of my life. I am sorry, but I will not sign any paper apologizing."

At that, Matt turned and walked out of the room.

After the turkey caper, the medical director and administration at Whitestone Hospital realized if they wanted to continue to get top-notch interns and residents, they'd better listen to the house staff.

When prospective medical students come to look over residency programs at any hospital, they always ask the house staff about the teaching program and whether they are happy with their surroundings. If the house staff is unhappy, next year's class would be a disaster in the "match."

The administration and executive medical staff members of Whitestone Hospital quickly decided to pay the interns and residents a small salary. Most of the hospitals around the country also started paying a minimal wage.

Before completing his second year of training, Matt was assigned to a tour of duty in the ER for six weeks—on duty for 24 hours and off for 24 hours.

In the daytime, the attending staff and resident staff are available in case a major catastrophe occurs. It is during the nighttime that much of the action develops and the house staff's responsibility increases.

If the first or second-year interns need help in the ER, there is a chain of command that they are to call. Private cases are taken care of by the attending doctors and unassigned cases by the residents.

At night when the attending doctor is called on the phone about one of his patients in the ER, he might make a few suggestions but often will tell the resident to handle the problem and have the patient see him the next day. If it is a potential surgical case for operating on that evening, the young surgical attending will often come in—the older surgical attending usually will tell the intern to call the chief surgical resident to see the case and then give him a call. On the ward cases, if the resident has a problem in the operating room, he has to call the responsible attending doctor.

There is an on-call room in the back of the ER that the junior assistant resident surgeon and first-year intern used for sleeping. It had a phone, a shower and the door had a bolt on it. That bolt came in handy on occasion.

The nursing staff who worked in the ER were some of the sharpest nurses in the hospital—their age and experience varied and their attitude in taking care of ER patients was efficiency plus. The night nurses who worked the eleven to seven shift had the most responsibility because, during that time, the availability of ancillary help was lowest.

The head nurse of that shift was a Ms. Steffi Pfeiffer, who had worked the "night owl" shift for years. Some residents resented her because she knew too much. She never hesitated to tell them what to do. One fact was known, she really knew how to mobilize the available help in the hospital if it was needed. She was a strict disciplinarian and knew more medicine than most of the interns.

The junior nurse on the "night owl" shift was a complete contrast to Steffi. Her name was Candy Goode. She was a 23-year-old, blue-eyed, blonde bombshell who was working at night so she could go to school in the daytime. She was about five feet, seven inches tall with long slender legs and thin hips that rotated appropriately and full-blossomed breasts that left nothing to the imagination, even in a tight-fitting nurse's uniform. Her big smile with pearl-white teeth and luscious lips could melt the heart of any virile male, including the younger single house staff doctors.

She had trained at Emory University in Atlanta. The combination of her beauty and southern drawl had a way of getting the resident staff over to see cases in the ER even in the wee hours of the morning. It wasn't the coffee in the ER that attracted the house staff—it was

Candy. Late at night the resident surgeons, after finishing operative cases, would often drop by to chat with Candy if the ER wasn't busy.

Candy had lots of opportunities for dates; dinner, sporting events, weekends in New York or Boston; you name it. However, she was not an easy one to get a date with. She was quite choosy and didn't want her lovelife to interfere with her studies.

Some of the single resident staff said they would be willing to give their right arm just to be able to "ring the bell" with Candy. A few of the attending staff tried to date her but were unsuccessful.

One of the busiest hand surgeons, Dr. Dubie, had propositioned her on more than one occasion. He told her that he'd leave his wife if she would cooperate appropriately. Candy wanted no part of him and told him off.

"If you'd stop wearing those L.L. Bean togs and dress up like a real man, I might be interested," she said. "All that money you've made off of hand surgery means beans to me. It's common knowledge that you charge too much! I'm sure you'd be a wimp in bed. I've got too much love to give to get involved with you. I'm also not interested in spending the rest of my life in shopping centers spending your money."

"No woman can talk to me like that and get away with it. I'm going to get you fired!" said Dr. Dubie.

"Go ahead. See if you can. I'll tell the hospital staff exactly the way you propositioned me. I might even embellish it a little with some intimate details. I'll also tell them how you harrassed me and threatened to have me fired. In fact, I think I'll talk to Steffi about our conversation."

The middle-aged hand surgeon thought for a minute, looked her in the eye to see if she meant business, and then said, "I'm sorry, Miss Goode. I guess I was trying to bridge the generation gap."

"Well, I'm not interested in bridging it with you," she replied. "You can take care of your ego and your pecker up in the North End. I believe it costs ten bucks."

Dr. Dubie got red in the face and stomped out of the ER. Candy had deflated his ego.

Not all the time on the eleven to seven shift was spent drinking coffee and conjuring up intimate thoughts about Candy. Major calamities occurred. Steffi and Candy could and did work as a superior efficient trauma team when they had to.

Matt got the ER rotation as a junior assistant resident in surgery in

May and June of his second year and was involved in an interesting surgical ER case during the eleven to seven night shift on a Friday night.

A large bank in one of the outlying communities was involved in a hold-up just before closing at 6 P.M. Quite a few of the banks stayed open late on Friday evening to get a competitive edge. Two ski-masked bank robbers entered the bank. One jumped over the counter so the tellers couldn't alert the police, while the other forced the personnel in the bank to lie on their stomachs as he held a sawed-off shotgun. They were professionals and well prepared, for the vault door was open.

They filled two large money bags with cash and then locked the bank personnel in a closet and took off. A getaway car showed up in front, driven by a female accomplice. A police officer saw them come out of the bank and told them to halt or he would fire. They ran toward the getaway car. He opened fire with his Smith and Wesson .38 revolver and called for help on his walkie-talkie. One of the bandits returned fire with a sawed-off shotgun. They sped away in their getaway car just as the police arrived in cruisers.

Evidently one of the bandits was hit by shots fired by the policeman because fresh, bright-red blood was found on the sidewalk in front of the bank. The police gave chase in their cruisers but lost them on the highways. When the detectives found the blood on the sidewalk, they notified all the surrounding hospitals of the bank robbery and the possibility that someone might show up in the ER with a bullet wound.

Sure enough, at 2:30 A.M., a woman called the ER at Whitestone Hospital and said that her husband had accidently shot himself in the neck while cleaning his gun. The ER notified the police of the call. Detectives in civilian clothes surrounded the ER area.

A car pulled up to the ER entrance and a young woman got out. A man staggered as he got out of the car and was immediately put on a stretcher.

Candy hollered for Matt and the intern for help. The man had difficulty breathing and was bleeding profusely from his mouth. He was quickly put in one of the big trauma rooms.

Matt noticed that the patient had a big hole on the left side of his cheek just above his jawbone and blood was pouring out. He put a T&A metal sucker into his mouth to suck the blood out. The patient was quite pale and weak from blood loss and didn't resist.

Matt put rubber gloves on and took a wad of gauze and packed it into the hole that was bleeding. He could feel that some of the teeth had been shattered.

"Candy, page Dr. Stetson, stat! Steffi, get an IV set up! We need to get some fluids into this guy. He's going to need a trach and he'll need blood. Alert the OR. We need to get him upstairs to find out where he's bleeding from. I'm going to hold my finger in his mouth to control ·the bleeding. Don't bite my finger off!" he hollered at the patient, "if you know what's good for you."

Stetson, the chief surgical resident, showed up just as they were pushing the patient into the elevator to take him to the operating room.

"Whatcha got, Matt?"

"Gunshot wound to the neck and cheek. He's gonna need a trach to control his airway and you're gonna have to look in his mouth to see where he's bleeding from."

Matt and Stetson took the patient directly into the operating room and anesthesia passed a tube down his throat to the lungs.

Once the cuff was blown up so the patient couldn't aspirate blood into his lungs, Stetson retracted the cheek with a metal retractor and took a good look at the bullet's point of entry and exit. It had penetrated through the cheek, shattering a couple of back upper molars—some of the fragments of the teeth were still in the mouth. A large bleeder was clamped and tied; blood and intravenous antibiotics were given, and the hole in the cheek patched up with fine silk sutures. He was lucky that the bullet didn't penetrate his brain.

The OR circulating nurse told Dr. Stetson that the detectives wanted him to save the fragments of the teeth found in the mouth. It turned out that the man that Stetson and Matt worked on was one of the bank robbers. He had stolen over $100,000 and stashed it away. The fragments of teeth and blood found on the sidewalk placed the patient at the scene of the crime. The bank robbers, including the female who drove the getaway car, were all caught.

The following day, everything returned to normal in the ER except that Dr. Kendall had a new first-year intern to work with for the following month. His name was David Ross, a six-foot five-inch former football player from the west coast. There were rumors spread by the nurses that he might be a homosexual. He hadn't dated any of the nurses.

When Candy met the Adonis-type male intern for the first time, she was obviously impressed by his handsome face and body. It was the first time that she showed any interest in any of the interns. Matt noticed that she started to wear provocative blouses and tight-fitting white pants. However, David didn't give her the time of day.

One evening, after David had been on duty for a week, Candy spoke to Matt.

"What's wrong with that intern friend of yours?" she asked. "Doesn't he have any hormones?"

"I hate to tell you this, Candy, I think he may be one of those. You know what I mean. That rumor that you nurses are spreading around may be true."

"Oh, what a shame!" replied Candy. "He's the first intern that I've seen that I might be willing to give up my family jewels for."

"I'd keep trying if you're still interested."

The next day, Matt mentioned to David that Candy had told him that she was interested in him and would like a date.

"She is quite pretty," replied David, nonchalantly.

"That's an understatement. She's built like a brick shithouse. If I was single, I'd be chasing her tail."

Three nights later, there was no action in the ER and David was catching some shut-eye in the on-call room.

Candy came up to Matt and asked where David was.

"He's getting some shut-eye in the on-call room."

"I have to see him. I want to ask him to go to a formal with me."

"Why don't you go back there and wake him up?"

"That's not a bad idea. Tell Steffi to cover me for a while."

Candy went back to the on-call room and quietly shut the door behind her. She put the bolt on and quickly took off all of her clothes. She gently got into the bed next to David, put her arms around him and placed her mouth on his. He responded to her kisses and as he woke up, she darted her tongue into his mouth. He didn't resist. She placed one of his hands on her breast. He realized who she was. He started to cooperate.

"Just relax, David," she said. "I want you to make love to me." He started to fondle her. She undid his belt and pulled down his trousers. She took his shorts off. She got on top of him and started rotating her buttocks. "I knew it would be like this," she said. "Am I making you happy?"

"Oh yes," replied David. "Very happy, Candy."

Two weeks later, Candy stopped working the night shift. It interfered with her lovelife. Candy and David got married three months later.

6

THE ER WAS MATT'S LAST ROTATION before his two-year residency was complete.

One evening, when he was on call in the ER, Dr. Stanley, the Chief of Surgery, came in to see a patient. Matt had ordered all the blood work and x-rays on the patient and they had been completed.

"Matt, what are you doing next year?" he asked.

"I'm thinking about going into surgery."

"Well, you've done a good job. I'll be glad to recommend you. However, you'd better make up your mind. Time is running out. We only have one slot left that's open."

"I'll get back to you tomorrow."

When he got home that evening, he and Nancy talked at length about their future. After much discussion and soul searching, they decided that he should talk to Dr. Stanley and apply for the surgical residency.

The program was unique in that one of the four chief residents would be selected to spend a year in training at Memorial Sloan Kettering Cancer Center in New York City. The New York trip was a sought-after position because of exposure to a large group of internationally known surgeons.

Matt worked hard when he got on the surgical service at Whitestone Hospital and enjoyed every minute. Now he felt he was doing what he wanted to do. Each surgical case was a challenge and it drove him to perform at his best.

The following year, Nancy got pregnant and they had their first child. It wasn't easy—Nancy was in labor for twenty-four hours and the obstetrician had to use forceps—the umbilical cord was wrapped around the baby's neck. Everything turned out all right.

Nancy delivered a beautiful, healthy, brown-eyed girl. They named her Betsy.

In his third year of surgical training, he was selected to make the New York trip. The problem was, once again, money. However, the rewards in New York City far outweighed the costs. Where would he get enough to finance his year in New York City? He heard about a medical education fund at Whitestone and decided to apply for a loan.

At the end of his third year of surgical training he and Nancy went to New York.

Matt soon found out that his duties as an assistant resident in surgery at Sloan Kettering Cancer Center were quite different from Whitestone Hospital. There was no emergency room to keep you up all night. Emergencies developed within the hospital but were different. On the head and neck service, respiratory obstruction was common and emergency tracheostomies were frequently done.

A major vascular calamity causing a carotid artery perforation in the neck happened occasionally. This was usually due to an infection or a weakness in the blood vessel wall caused by tumor or radiation damage. During the time Dr. Kendall was on the head and neck service, one of Dr. Hayes' patients, an Arab, was staying at the Waldorf Astoria after his radical neck surgery. He developed an infection. One day, as he got off the elevator in the main lobby of the hotel, he blew his carotid blood vessel in his neck, and died on the spot. The afternoon newspaper carried a story that a prominent Arab sheik had been shot in the head and died within minutes in the lobby of the hotel. The article stated, "Blood splattered all over the rugs," evincing not only the fallibility of the human body, but of human journalists as well.

Radical surgery was the main method of treating cancer in the 1950s. If the cancer could be cut out before it spread, the theory was that the patient could be cured. Patients from all walks of life came to Memorial Sloan Kettering Cancer Center. Some individuals, from distant foreign countries, would arrive with a tag pinned to their shirt with the hospital's name on it. Famous show-biz people and scores of businessmen, all desperate, came for help.

One of the first services Matt rotated through was the GYN service, run by Dr. Alexander Hart, one of the giants in the radical surgical approach to the treatment of cancer. He was an international authority on the surgical treatment of pancreatic, liver, and pelvic tumors and was particularly noted for doing total pelvic exenterations, such as the removal of multiple organs involved with cancer of the cervix, bladder, and rectum.

Colostomies (bringing the opening of the bowel onto the abdominal wall) were performed and new bladders were made (reimplantation of the ureters that drain the water from the kidneys). The blood loss was quite large in some of these operations, creating a challenge for the surgeon and the anesthesiologist. It was the first time Matt saw intravenous access (IVs placed in both arms and the use of a hand pump to maintain blood volume) so the patient wouldn't go into shock.

James Ewing Hospital was the large city hospital attached to the Memorial Sloan Kettering Hospital, and it was at Ewing that resident surgeons did most of their surgery. Usually they would rotate through the private service first, watching and assisting the experts, and then were assigned to the ward service at James Ewing, where they would do surgery under supervision. It was here that the responsibility of the total care of the patient came to rest on the young surgical resident's shoulders.

Four weeks after being on the gynecological service at James Ewing Hospital, Matt was involved in an unusual case. He had assisted one of the senior surgical residents on a radical hysterectomy and lymphadenectomy. He then went with the patient to the recovery room.

When they reached the recovery room the woman's vital signs—blood pressure and pulse—were all normal. The anesthesiologist then left the recovery room. As Matt was writing postoperative orders for the patient, the recovery room nurse called him and said, "I don't like the looks of this patient."

"What's wrong?"

"Her pulse is rapid. She's cold and clammy and her blood pressure is dropping. How did everything go with the operation?"

"It was kind of wet. Not the best. She got five units of blood. Why don't you speed up the blood and order a couple of more units."

Matt continued to write orders and then spoke to the recovery room nurse. "Page the chief resident and tell him I want him to come back and take a look at her." The extra blood arrived and was started. About five minutes later, the recovery room nurse spoke up again and said the patient's pressure had dropped to 70/0 with a pulse of 160.

Matt went to the patient's bed and pulled the sheets off and between her legs he saw a large pool of blood. She obviously had blown a large blood vessel inside her abdomen and was bleeding through the vagina. At that point, her blood pressure dropped out of sight and she went into cardiac arrest.

"Get help. Now!" he hollered at the nurse. He was in a dilemma as to whether he should open the chest and try heart massage or attempt to stop the bleeding coming through the vagina.

"Help. Help!" hollered the recovery room nurse to the other nurses in the room. "Put a stat page in for Dr. Bonson."

Matt grabbed a surgical instrument set. It would be useless to open the chest and massage the heart if she had a large hole in an artery or vein. If he squeezed the heart, he would just be pumping more blood out of her system.

He decided to open the belly incision. He took a heavy scissors and rapidly cut through the abdominal sutures. Her lower belly was filled with blood. He scooped the blood out quickly and took a large Kelly clamp and clamped the left iliac vein that looked like it had a hole in it. He packed the vein and told one of the recovery room nurses to hold pressure on the packs.

Matt felt only a vague distress—he was too much within the problem to feel emotion. He took a scalpel and made an incision in the left chest, he reached in and took the heart in the palm of his hand and started to squeeze. Just then, the anesthesiologist and the chief surgical resident arrived. An endotracheal tube was rapidly passed into her lungs for oxygenation and more blood was pumped into her veins. Her blood volume was rapidly replaced and suddenly her heartbeat came back. The patient was rushed back into the operating room. The leaking blood vessel in the pelvis was sutured and tied and the abdomen and chest wounds were closed.

Except for some latent kidney problems and a longer stay in the hospital, the patient survived and was able to walk out of the hospital. Luckily, she didn't have any brain damage. She wasn't thrilled with the big scar on her chest that had been made to massage her heart, but she was alive.

One week before completing his surgical rotation at Memorial Sloan Kettering Cancer Center, Matt was called to the chief surgeon's office.

"Matt, we've enjoyed having you with us here in New York. We'd like you to come back and take a fellowship in cancer. You've done a tremendous job! Our attending staff is impressed with your surgical skills."

"Thanks. I'll have to give it some thought."

"It's an opportunity of a lifetime," said the Chief.

"I know, but I'd better discuss it with my wife."

7

IN JULY, after completing his one-year surgical residency training in New York City, Matt returned to Whitestone Hospital to become one of the chief resident surgeons. His first assignment was on the South Surgical Service with Dr. Phillip McBratney as his chief attending.

It was standard procedure for the chief resident surgeon and the chief attending surgeon to meet each morning to see and discuss all the sick patients before going into the operating room. They would do hands-on examinations as they made their walking surgical rounds. Usually the intern or first-year surgical resident presented the pertinent points of the history and any diagnostic tests that needed to be discussed, such as blood work or x-rays.

He soon found out that Dr. McBratney had an unpredictable dry sense of humor. His greetings in the morning were often inquisitive and had a purpose.

"What trouble did you boys get into last night?"

Matt's answer was cautious because Dr. McBratney was known to have a temper if things didn't go right.

"We had two difficult, but interesting cases last night."

"Well, don't keep me in suspense. Tell me about it."

"We had an elderly alcoholic man come in with a big, bulging mass in his lower abdomen and right groin at around 6 P.M. He had been drinking quite a bit and was vomiting. Dr. Thompson, one of our assistant surgical residents, saw him in the emergency room and thought he might have a strangulated hernia. He tried to reduce the hernia in the emergency room by gently pressing on the mass but the patient didn't cooperate."

"What sort of work-up did Thompson do?"

"A good history was not obtainable because the patient was drunk.

Physical exam showed a large mass in the right groin that was tender to touch. Abdomen was slightly distended and bowel sounds were hyperactive. We did a white blood count, which was elevated, and a flat plate and erect x-ray of the abdomen to see if there was any obstruction of the bowel or free air."

"What did the x-ray show?"

"Distended large and small bowel. The radiologist called it a bowel obstruction."

"Did anyone do a rectal exam?"

"Yes. Normal digital exam."

"How sick did the patient look?"

"Extremely."

"Well, did you put a tube down his stomach to help decompress the bowel to get the air out and book him in the operating room?"

"Yes. But the OR was backed up. Everybody was calling their case an emergency and they all wanted priority."

"Did anesthesia call in their extra team to help out?"

"Not immediately," replied Matt. "Not until Dr. MacDuffie insisted that his fractured hip case be done stat."

"Did you challenge him? You had a more life-threatening situation with a possible strangulated bowel. His case was not life-threatening."

"I tried to tell him that, but he wouldn't listen. Besides, I'm only a resident and he's a senior attending."

Dr. McBratney looked up at the ceiling. He blew out a deep breath. "What did the anesthesiologist say? Did he challenge MacDuffie?"

"No. He didn't say anything. We finally got into the OR at around 10:00 P.M."

"That figures! What was your preoperative diagnosis?"

"I wasn't convinced it was a hernia. I knew the patient was very sick and needed to be operated on. His belly was tense. He was definitely obstructed."

"What did your junior resident, Dr. Thompson, think?"

"He thought it was a strangulated hernia."

"What sort of incision did you make?"

"The assistant resident wanted to make an incision directly over the mass."

"Did you let him do the case?"

"No."

"Good," said McBratney. "When in doubt, you have to wield the knife. You're the responsible surgeon."

"We made the incision of indecision—a lower right rectus abdominal incision and there was a big mass in the right gutter of the abdomen. There wasn't any pus. There was also a hernia present."

"Well, what did you do? What were your thoughts?"

"At first I thought we had a ruptured appendix with a walled off abscess but it didn't look like that. I did a little sharp dissection and the appendix looked normal. It looked like and felt like a right colon cancer similar to a few cases I had seen in New York. I was worried because he didn't have a bowel cleansing prep and we might get spillage. I was also worried about Crohn's disease—inflammatory disease of the bowel. I thought he might have a problem like President Eisenhower had. The bowel was distended."

"OK, doctor, you've got me in suspense. One more question. Did you consult with your attending surgeon on call?"

"Not really. We were there and we had to act."

"Did you try to call him?"

"Yes and he said to call him back if we had a problem with the surgery. I decided to do a right hemicolectomy. We took the mass and the right side of the colon out. When we opened the specimen we found that the patient had a cancer of the proximal colon—the cecum."

"Did you do a colostomy or consider a cecostomy to let the gas out of the distended bowel?"

"No. The bowel looked OK and the tube to decompress the bowel had traveled and was doing its job. We also gave him intravenous antibiotics."

"How's he doing?"

"OK so far."

"Well, you can argue the management of that case in any direction you want. If he does OK, you made the right decision. Your logic wasn't bad. Anything else happen last night?"

"Yes. It's something I don't like and I want to discuss it."

"This sounds serious."

"It is! We finished that first case at 1 A.M. and I was called to the emergency room to see another abdomen at 2 A.M. The patient was a seventy-three-year-old man with severe back pain. I've been waiting to see a patient like this since that trip I made to Houston, Texas to watch DeBakey work. The patient had a pulsating mass in his abdomen and I recognized that he might have a leaking aneurysm. I felt that one of the large blood vessels in his belly had ruptured. I alerted the operating room and blood bank and did a stat I.V.P. It showed the ureters pushed laterally by a large mass. I quickly put two large intravenous lines in for blood replacement during surgery and then I called the attending on the Ward Service, Dr. Maurice, to come in and assist with the operation. He met me in the scrub room at 5 A.M. We scrubbed, anesthesia put the patient out and the abdomen was prepped. The scrub nurse handed the knife to me, and Dr. Maurice said, 'I'll be doing this operation.'

"I challenged him. 'This is a ward patient, Dr. Maurice.'

'We haven't had any survivors of leaking aneurysms in this hospital,' he replied, 'I'll take the scalpel.' "

"What did you do?" asked McBratney.

"He was the boss. What could I do? We had to save the patient's life, so I decided I would do my best to help him. He made a big abdominal incision and when we got into the abdomen, there was free blood in the cavity spreading rapidly around the tissues and distending the bowel.

"Dr. Maurice dissected and freed up the tissue around the ruptured aorta. He took a large vascular clamp and applied it gently on the big blood vessel. The blood vessel was brittle, as fragile as egg shells. It crumbled under the pressure and ruptured completely. The patient rapidly bled out and died within minutes."

"Goddamn it," said Dr. McBratney. "That jerk is going to be the death of me!" He thought for a moment. "Well, Matt, I'll talk to Dr. Maurice. That will be the last time he does that to one of my residents. Next time you're to call me. That was a ward case and I'm the boss. However, you're better off in the long run you didn't do that one."

"Well, I couldn't have screwed it up any worse than he did."

Dr. McBratney smiled. "I'm inclined to agree with you." He liked his young chief resident surgeon.

Before the end of his chief surgical residency year, Matt was involved with a general surgeon, Dr. Jack Diamond, and a young excellent Chinese vascular surgeon in the first successful repair of a ruptured aortic aneurysm at Whitestone Hospital. Theirs was the first patient to come out of the operating room alive after that type of operation.

One of the chief resident surgeon's jobs is to learn to deal with anything that arrives at the emergency room door. When things slowed down in the operating room, Matt hung out in the emergency room at night looking for action.

Karen, the night nursing supervisor, stopped Matt one night as he walked through the ER. "Dr. Kendall, will you help pronounce a patient for us? He was just brought in by ambulance from a motel and it looks like it might be a coroner's case."

"What happened?"

"Evidently, this guy was with his wife at one of those love motels and died suddenly. The EMTs had to drag him out of one of those heart-shaped love tubs."

"You mean he drowned?"

"We don't know," said Karen.

"Did his wife come in with him?"

"Yes, she's in the room. She's pretty broken up."

"I suppose I've got to ask her some questions."

"She's not coherent," said Karen. "Anyway, go in there and pronounce him."

"OK."

Matt went into the room where the body was. The body lying on the stretcher was fully dressed in a yellow silk jacket with fancy trousers and black shoes. He had no respirations, no corneal reflex, his color was ashen, and rigor mortis was setting in.

"I'm sorry I have to tell you that your husband is dead."

The woman let out a wail, hearing what she already knew. Tears began rolling down her cheeks as she held her hands together in a prayer fashion, rocking to and fro.

"I know this is rough. But you're not alone. We can call one of our clergy to talk to you if you'd like. What was his religion?"

"Catholic," said the woman, collecting herself. "But don't call the priest. Not just yet."

"I can order a tranquilizer for you if you think you might need one."

"No, I'll be all right as soon as I collect my thoughts."

"We'll need to know his full name, age, address and his insurance."

"I can give you most of that information."

"The coroner is also going to want to ask you some questions, since you were the last one to see him alive."

"Oh, no, I can't do that," she replied. "I'm in no condition for that."

Matt looked at her more closely. She was an attractive blonde about five feet, seven inches tall, maybe 35 years old, wearing an expensive pink suit, white spiked heels, with a beautiful tan. She looked quite a bit younger than the man laid out on the stretcher.

"Perhaps you can answer some questions for me. The coroner may accept that."

"I think that might be better," she said.

"What motel were you at?"

"The Embassy Motel down on the turnpike. We were relaxing in one of those love tubs, when he suddenly got chest pain and slumped over. I tried to pull him out of the tub but he was too heavy for me.

"I ran to the phone and called the front desk to get a doctor or an ambulance. Then I ran back to the tub. He was face down in the water. I grabbed his hair and pulled his face out of the water and I slapped him hard, trying to wake him. He had been drinking but not so much that I thought he'd pass out.

"Finally, a bellboy arrived and helped me pull him out of the tub and put him on the floor. He pushed and pounded on his chest. There was no response. The bellboy said, 'He ain't gonna make it,' but he kept pushing on his chest.

"The motel office called for an ambulance and I went into the bedroom and got dressed. There wasn't anything more I could do. My heart was pounding. I felt sick. I think I was in shock."

"How old was he?" asked Matt.

"He was 58."

"He had his clothes on when he arrived here. How did that happen?"

"The EMTs arrived and they tried everything they could to resuscitate him, but nothing worked. He was dead. They helped me put some clothes on him and then they transported him to the hospital."

"Do you have any children?"

"No," she said. "I'm single. He's married and has two children."

"That could be a little bit awkward, since this will be a coroner's case. There will be an inquiry."

"Oh, no. I can't do that. I don't want to face his wife."

"Well, talk to the coroner then," said Matt. "Maybe when his wife reads the report she won't want to see you. But then again, maybe she will."

"I think I'll take a month's vacation in Florida," replied the woman.

"I think that's what I'd do," said Matt, and with that he walked out of the room.

8

In the spring, as Dr. Kendall was completing his surgical residency at Whitestone, he and his wife discussed going back to New York City. They were still broke, living at poverty level, and had a daughter and a son to feed and clothe. They were undecided as to what they should do.

"It would be good for your practice if we could afford it," said his wife.

"I know," said Matt. "It could help make us independent. Maybe I can apply for a National Cancer Institute Fellowship. They pay some money. Are you ready for the city—the Big Apple?"

"I'm willing to give it a try," replied Nancy.

He decided to apply for a fellowship at Memorial Sloan Kettering Cancer Institute and several weeks later, he got a letter of acceptance.

The time quickly arrived for the move to New York.

The term "U-Haul-It," means exactly what it says. When someone has to move from one place to another, possessions accumulated need to be transferred. Not all belongings are worthy of transfer but they may have sentimental value.

Matt and Nancy had no money for moving expenses. They were unable to afford a moving van so they explored their options, and finally went to a truck and trailer rental company and rented a large trailer. Getting the trailer is the easy part. The hard part is putting the furniture and other possessions into the trailer and hoping that the jalopy you drive can pull the trailer.

There's a cooperative effort in the educational underground. "You help me and I'll help you." Money is not transferred in the deal and what you get is a sore back and aching shoulders.

One method is to buy a six-pack of beer, get some food together, and find a couple of young doctors who are willing to help you load the trailer. That's helpful at the departing end of the deal. Unfortunately, when you get to your destination, you're on your own.

Two young interns at Whitestone Hospital volunteered to help Matt load the trailer as long as the beer continued to flow.

"What are you moving this dilapidated, old, heavyweight sofa for? It looks like it ought to be in the dump," said one of the interns.

"Because I don't know where the dump is in New York City," he replied. "Otherwise, I would go there and find one to take its place."

"Just walk down some of the lower east side alleyways and there are plenty of dilapidated sofas you can use. You might find a few stiffs there too! You're crazy going to New York," he replied.

"Thanks for your encouragement," said Matt. "It makes me feel so good."

The car and trailer were loaded on a Saturday morning, and the plan was to drive to New York City on Sunday.

There were two more little problems that had to be taken care of properly. There were now two little indians in their brood—Betsy, who was three-and-a-half years old, quite talkative, and very opinionated. Matt said that she took after her mother and Nancy made no heritage claims. "She really takes after you, Matt."

Mike, the youngest addition, was eighteen months old and was a real problem to take care of because he had a milk intolerance and had to be fed special food. He also had eczema and was constantly itching and scratching. They were two great active kids, however, and a joy to the family when they were good. They also had to be loaded into the car for the trip to New York City. Nancy and Matt had said a prayer hoping they might sleep on the trip.

Matt told Nancy to withdraw two hundred dollars out of their bank account so if they needed money, they'd have it. He had sold his set of golf clubs to a young attending at the hospital and had another $100 in his pocket. He purposely didn't tell Nancy about the extra $100.

Before they left Sunday morning, Nancy cooked a big breakfast.

"I don't know about you, but my back aches already," said Nancy, as they started down the main highway heading toward New York City.

"Well, my back isn't exactly in great shape either," replied Matt.

He felt he was sparring with her to see which one of them had contributed the most so far. They usually had a battle royal every time they moved, and it ended up being a tearful experience and then later a reconciliation.

Arguments began as the old 1939 Dodge sedan struggled to pull the trailer. The car had no air conditioning. The air conditioning came from the hole in the floorboard just below the driver. If there was water on the highway, a nice little dirty splatter would compliment your clothes. The best part of the car was the radio. It could be turned up loud.

Fifteen minutes after heading for New York on the four-lane highway, Betsy spoke up.

"When are we going to be there, Daddy?"

"Just relax Betsy, we've just started down the road. Play with your dolly."

"I don't want to play with my dolly. I want to see what's going on."

Betsy crawled up and strained to look between Nancy and Matt.

"Try to keep that one occupied, if you please?" said Matt as he looked over at Nancy. "I've got my hands full trying to drive this jalopy."

"I'll try," said Nancy. "I've got a feeling in the pit of my stomach that we may have bitten off more than we can chew with this trip."

"Well, don't jinx the trip before we get started," said Matt.

Nancy turned to Betsy and said, "Why don't you look at the pictures in that pretty book that I gave you to look at?"

Betsy just looked up at Nancy with an inquisitive glance and said, "No!"

After a short while, Betsy laid back on a pillow and started to close her eyes.

"Thank goodness!" said Nancy.

As they rode along in the old workhorse of a car they felt like bride and groom, except for the kids, because of the number of cars and trucks honking their horns at them. The rubbernecking and smiles on their faces didn't help the situation. The honking was because the car could only do forty miles an hour hauling the heavy trailer. Driving forty miles an hour on an interstate highway is like waiting for a catastrophe to happen.

Well, it happened. As they approached Stamford, Connecticut, the traffic going into the city increased and suddenly the poor old Dodge had had it. It had trouble pulling the trailer. No matter how hard Matt pushed on the accelerator, the forward speed decreased. He started to edge the car over to the side of the road. A thumping sound began to get louder and louder and louder behind the car as he slowed down. He knew he had big trouble. He eased the car over to the curb and stopped it. Nancy, who had dozed off, suddenly woke up from her nap.

"What are you stopping for?"

"Because the car won't go forward. That's why! Don't ask stupid questions!" He got out of the car and surveyed the problem. A tire on the trailer was flat.

"What do we do now?" asked Nancy.

"I hate to tell you. We've got to unload the trailer in order to put a new tire on. We don't have a spare."

"That's great. Why don't we detach the trailer and leave this junk here?" said Nancy as she started to cry.

"Might not be a bad idea. Except that I signed papers that makes me responsible for the trailer. I'll walk down the road to a gas station and get a tire."

"Do you have any money?"

"Enough to get a tire. That tire on the trailer looks like it's the same size tire as the car. Maybe I can use our spare tire that's in the trunk."

"Maybe not, too! Don't forget, we filled the trunk with boxes," said Nancy.

"We'll just have to unload it then, to get to the tire."

He opened the trunk and started to unload all the odds and ends out onto the grass. The temperature was 100°. They unloaded the trunk and found a spare tire. They also found the six-pack of beer he had hidden there before they started on the trip.

"I don't drink," said Nancy, "but I'll take one of those."

It took them another hour to unload the trailer. When they got the trailer unloaded, up in front in an enclosed compartment was a spare tire. "Damn!" said Matt as he changed the tire. When he finished, they had to reload the trailer and the trunk of the car. That took another hour.

Luckily for Matt and Nancy, the two kids slept in the car while they changed the tire. Betsy woke up just as they were ready to move back out on the highway.

"I need to go to the bathroom, Mommy," she said.

"Well, I guess we have to take a little walk and go over there in the bushes," said Nancy.

"I don't like going to the bathroom in the bushes," replied Betsy.

Finally, they were back on the road again heading for the Big Apple.

They each had a second beer. A strange silence prevailed so Matt put the car radio back on and turned the volume up.

"This surgical residency had better be worth it," said Nancy, "because it certainly is starting out in an ominous way."

"I don't want to hear any more of that," he said as he turned the volume of the radio up still further.

They continued to chug along, getting closer to the city. They finally saw the sign indicating they were entering New York state. The toll booths reminded them that their financial resources were depleting.

They finally got on the Hutchinson River Parkway.

"I think we have to go toward the George Washington Bridge if we want to get to lower Manhattan."

"That takes you into Jersey," said Nancy.

"I know, but I don't think they allow trailers to go down the East River Drive. They won't let you cross the Triborough Bridge with a trailer."

"How can we get to lower Manhattan with the trailer then?" Nancy asked.

"We have to head for the George Washington Bridge. I think we have to go up around 165th Street and head down the West Side. Get out that Mobil map in the glove compartment."

"That won't tell you if they allow trailers on the East River Drive!"

"Thank you," Matt curtly replied. The back of his neck was getting red. He contemplated strangling his wife. They decided to head toward the George Washington Bridge and then go down toward 68th Street by going through the middle of town.

"That way will take us right through Harlem," said Nancy. "What if we get another flat tire?"

"You're so optimistic. If we get another flat tire, I'll give you a heavy wrench to defend yourself. I'll watch the kids. Besides, who would want to steal this junk anyway?"

Nancy started to cry. Things seemed to be getting worse—silence prevailed.

They finally arrived at 68th and York on the East Side. As one could have predicted, there were no available parking spaces. "What do we do now?" asked Nancy. "We can't leave this car and trailer in the middle of the road."

"Find a parking space as close to our apartment as possible so we don't break our backs. We can unload this crap anytime," replied Matt.

They drove up and down the street looking for a parking space. There weren't any available. Fortunately, it was a hot Sunday and people were still going to the local beaches. After driving around for what seemed like an eternity, looking like a couple of gypsies in the middle of the Sahara Desert, a parking place opened up near the apartment. They grabbed it.

"I'll check in at the hospital and get the keys to the apartment," said Matt. "You watch the car and the kids."

He came back with the keys and when they got to their new apartment on the eleventh floor there were voices coming from inside. When they opened the door, packed boxes were all over the place. A resident, who had completed his fellowship, was there with his wife and a three-year-old boy.

"Where the hell have you been?" asked the young doctor.

"Driving to the Big Apple," said Matt.

"Well, if you help us unload the apartment you'll have a place to put your furniture."

Matt thought for a minute. The guy looked fairly strong. They couldn't move in without them out of there and his back was aching. "I'll do it a load for a load," Matt said.

"What do you mean?" he asked.

"We'll bring a load of yours down and then you'll help us bring a load of ours up."

The young doctor smiled. "It's a bargain."

The four of them spent three hours loading and unloading. Finally, the job was done. Matt and Nancy were totally exhausted. They finished the last beer from the six-pack.

"Next time we move, I'm going to buy two six-packs," said Matt.

"I'll vote for that!" replied Nancy.

Living in New York City is very expensive. Matt's income for supporting himself, his wife, his daughter Betsy, and son Mike, was barely enough for them to live on so he had to find some way to supplement his income.

Nancy was a nurse, so she decided she would work one night a week at New York Hospital while he babysat. He would moonlight one night a week at Manhattan General Hospital on the lower East Side, working as a surgical house officer, starting intravenous feedings, doing catheterizations, and scrubbing on evening emergency operations.

The night supervisor at Manhattan General Hospital, Annie Jones, was a pleasure to work with. One night as Matt came in, she briefed him on a few complex cases the attending surgeons wanted him to see.

"Any real sick ones?"

"A couple. Dr. Veilleux wants you to look at Mr. Casey, an elderly man, who came in around 4:30. He's doubled up with abdominal pain, has a fever, elevated white count, and is getting progressively worse."

"What's he got, an appendix?"

"He had his appendix out thirty years ago by a surgeon called One-Inch Lynch."

"Who's One-Inch Lynch? What do you know about him?"

"Well, he's dead now. He was a hotshot Park Avenue surgeon who made his reputation by taking out the appendix through a one-inch incision in the right lower quadrant. The women liked him because he never left a big scar on their belly. I heard some of his patients were showgirls who worked on 52nd Street."

"Nice clientele. Where's the patient?"

"He's up on five."

Matt went up and examined the patient and found tenderness in the right lower quadrant of his abdomen. He put pressure over the abdominal wall and quickly released it, creating some rebound pressure, which in turn created pain. Bowel sounds were quiet.

"He's sick, all right," Matt said to the floor nurse. "Order a flat plate and erect x-ray of the belly to see if he's perforated a viscus or is obstructed. Also notify his surgeon that he needs to be put on the operating schedule for tonight."

"What do you think it is? It certainly can't be his appendix."

"I don't know, not unless he's grown another one. My exam reveals he has impending peritonitis—if he doesn't already have it. He's really sick! He needs a look inside. Have him typed and cross-matched for blood. Get me a saline IV and I'll start an intravenous. Notify his family that he's in trouble and get the permission slip signed."

Matt examined four more patients and ordered tests but most were routine—nothing that couldn't wait.

"So what else is going on upstairs?" he asked.

"Well, Dr. Gold, one of our ENT plastic surgeons, asked me if I'd have you check one of his nose jobs that he did today."

"Oh, come on. Let him take care of his own nose bobs. That's not in my contract."

"There's no one covering the ENT service tonight," said Annie, "and you're it."

"That's great. Do I get a raise if I see the patient?"

"No. But you'll make me happy and you could help a sick young lady."

"Let's go see her, then. I want you to be happy."

Annie and Matt took the elevator to the operating room floor and walked into the recovery room.

Sitting bolt upright in the bed was a sixteen-year-old girl who had just vomited a great deal of bright red blood and mucous. Both of her eyes were swollen shut and both cheeks were black and blue from extravasation of blood in the tissues. She looked like someone had hit her with a baseball bat. Matt took a tongue blade and looked down her throat. He could see some bright red blood running down the back. He took her pulse. It was rapid (140) and she looked pale.

He walked away from the bed and said to Annie, "He calls this a nose job? She looks like she's been in a street fight in Brooklyn. We'll have to start an intravenous on her. Does she have any blood on call?"

"No," replied Annie.

"Well, type and cross-match her for three units of blood—stat! Notify Dr. Gold about the problem. Find out if there is anything else I should know about her. Did her surgeon have any problems in the operating room? Was there an accident?"

"Not that I know about," said Annie. "There's one thing, though. She has a twin sister who had a nose job done at the same time in the next operating room. He was bobbing both of their noses, but the other one's all right. Her mother wanted the twins to look alike and to go into show business."

"Wonderful! Doing nose jobs on twins so you can match them up for a television producer? Well, I have news for mom—the one with the bleeding is not going to have the same nose as her sister. Order a hematocrit to see how much blood she's lost and stat it. Give me a call when you get the results. Any other lovely little problems for this evening?" Matt asked, smiling at Annie.

"Yes, just one more. She's down in the emergency room."

"What surprise do you have for me there?"

"Well, as you know, this hospital is unionized," said Annie, with some trepidation, "and the wife of the union president is down there with a speck of dirt in her eye. I think she needs it washed out."

"You can do that."

"Of course I can. But she's a bitch on wheels and she wants the chief resident to do it. You're the man."

"Thanks a lot."

Annie went with Matt to the emergency room. Sitting on the side of an examining table was an obese woman in her sixties wearing a full length mink coat.

"Where have you been?" she hollered as Matt walked into the room.

"Seeing sick patients," he replied.

"Well, my husband is the head of the union of this hospital and I plan to tell him how long I had to wait."

"That's your privilege. What's your problem?"

"My right eye hurts and I think I got a piece of dirt in it."

"Sit over here so I can get a look." Matt gestured the woman over to the optical equipment. She lurched off the exam table and motioned Annie to help her.

Matt took a Q-tip and rolled her upper eyelid up. He focused the bright light on the cornea of her eye.

"I'm going to put a few drops in your eye, Mrs. Domkowski. Do you have any allergies?"

"Not that I know of," she replied.

He put some fluorescene dye into her eye and then focused the light. There was a minute foreign body right over the center of the lens.

"Mrs. Domkowski, you have a foreign body that's slightly embedded right over the center of the lens of your right eye."

"Well, take it out," she yelled. "It hurts!"

"I'm sorry, I'm not an eye doctor. I'll put some medication in the eye that will take the pain away and some antibiotics to prevent infection and you can see your eye man in the morning."

"Why can't you take it out?" she asked.

"Because I'm not qualified. I don't want to make a permanent scratch on your lens."

"Oh, so all this flattery I've heard about young Dr. Kendall is a bunch of crap."

"Perhaps," he said. "But whatever you've heard about me won't turn me into an eye specialist. You've heard my advice. Take it or leave it."

Annie Jones, hearing the conversation, tried to placate Mrs. Domkowski. "Dr. Kendall is one of our best doctors," she said. "We'll have one of our eye men see you first thing in the morning. I'm sure you'll be all right."

"He's rude and shouldn't be working here," said Mrs. Domkowski.

"Maybe we'll be able to get an eye man to come in and see you tonight," Annie suggested.

"Not likely," said Matt as he smiled.

"They'd better get an eye man in here tonight or he'll be fired off the staff," screamed the patient.

"Good luck with those ophthalmologists on call, Annie," Matt snickered.

"You haven't heard the end of this, Dr. Kendall," said Mrs. Domkowski.

"For now I have," he said. "I'm going up to the x-ray department to look at the flat plate on that guy with the acute belly pain."

Matt went to the x-ray department. The cecum at the beginning of the large bowel in the lower right quadrant of the abdomen was dilated and there were signs of early obstruction, indicating that he needed to be operated on promptly.

He told the nurses to start the patient on intravenous antibiotics and called Annie and told her to get the anesthesia team in. The patient was getting worse.

He then went to the recovery room and saw the sick twin. She was still bleeding. Her pulse was rapid and she looked pale. Her hematocrit was down to 25. He decided to start a blood transfusion.

"Did you get Dr. Gold?" he asked Annie.

"No. His answering service is trying to find him."

"Is there anybody covering him?"

"I doubt it," she replied. "He usually doesn't have any complications."

"Well he's got one now and he'd better get his ass in here. Tell that answering service it's an emergency. Run the two units of blood in rapidly and when they're finished do another hematocrit to see where we stand with the bleeding."

"Dr. Kendall, Dr. Kendall, wanted in the operating room," a stern voice announced over the page system.

"I guess Dr. Veilleux finally got in here." He met the doctor in the locker room of the doctor's lounge.

"What have we got here?" Dr. Veilleux asked.

"I don't know, it's a weirdo. His appendix is out. His abdomen is distended, there's no bowel sounds and he's got rebound. He could have a perforated cancer of the cecum. Either way, he's really sick and needs to be explored. I started intravenous antibiotics."

Both doctors scrubbed, and entered the operating room.

"Why don't you do the honors?" suggested Dr. Veilleux. "I'll assist you."

"OK," Matt replied, always eager to operate.

"What kind of an incision are you going to make?" asked Dr. Veilleux.

"A lower right rectus."

"Sounds like a good idea."

After prepping the abdominal wall, draping it with sterile sheets, and getting the go-ahead to start from anesthesia, Matt compressed the scalpel against the lower abdominal wall, sharply cutting through the skin. Clamps were applied to the bleeders and they were tied with silk. The peritoneum was picked up with Kelly clamps and the belly opened. Foul-smelling pus evacuated from the abdomen. Most of it seemed to be located in the right lower quadrant.

"We'll need more relaxation," Dr. Kendall remarked to the anesthesiologist, as he had Dr. Veilleux pull the retractors against the abdominal wall to see the right colon.

Using the Metzenbaum dissecting scissors he sharply incised the area near the beginning of the large bowel. He saw the right ureter in the back of the abdomen as it came from the right kidney underneath the bowel. "We don't want to cut that," said Matt. Then he saw what he thought was impossible. "Well, look at what we have here," he said, as he gently brought out and removed a fat, worm-like structure from behind the bowel. "This is one appendix that One-Inch Lynch didn't get. I wonder what he charged for that operation? No wonder he used a one-inch incision on that case. We'll have to use quite a few drains on this one." He put Penrose drains in place and rapidly closed the belly.

After taking a quick shower he went back to see the sick twin. She looked worse. He ordered two more units of blood.

"Get Dr. Gold," he told Annie. "I've got to talk to him. This girl is fading, and unless he wants to be the first plastic surgeon responsible for a nose-job fatality, he'd better get his ass in here."

It was one in the morning. Annie finally got Dr. Gold on the phone. He was at a cocktail party out on the island and sounded like he had had a few drinks. Before Matt could say anything, Dr. Gold shouted, "Why the hell are you bothering me at this hour, Kendall?"

"Because you have a real sick patient," he replied.

"What's the problem?"

"One of the twins you operated on this morning has continued to bleed since your operation."

"How do you know?"

"I looked in the back of her throat. She has bright red blood running down the back of her throat and she's vomiting. She's got a rapid pulse and blood studies show she's continued to bleed. Her hematocrit dropped to twenty-five."

"This has never happened to me before," said Gold, sounding hurt. "Have you given her blood?"

"She's had three units. I think you should come in right away and see her."

"I'm not too eager to do that," he replied. "I'd have to take that big dressing down on her face and put in a posterior pack. She'd be a mess."

"She's already a mess. Her problem is persistent bleeding. Call a cab, and get over here."

"Give her some more blood and call me back in an hour."

Matt thought of finding out where Gold was, driving there, and putting him in the kind of shape his patient was in. He took a deep breath. Then another. Dr. Gold was evading his responsibility.

"You'd better order three more units of blood," he told Annie. "Also keep her in the recovery room. Have them set up a trach set and keep me informed."

At 3:30 A.M. he ordered another hematocrit. It came back 22. She was still bleeding and vomiting blood. He called Dr. Gold again.

"Dr. Gold, you have to come in and see your patient! She's dying. I can't replace her blood fast enough and she may need a trach."

"All right, all right, Doctor. Calm down! Alert the operating room and anesthesia. I'll be right in." He sounded agitated and disgusted.

"Right in" turned out to be one hour later. It was now 4:30 A.M. Matt met Dr. Gold in the recovery room.

"God, she's a mess," exclaimed Dr. Gold. "Why didn't you call me sooner?"

"We've been calling you since 8 P.M. Annie Jones will verify that."

"Yes, yes," he replied.

"I think you're going to have to trach her under local anesthesia because the anesthesiologist won't be able to get a tube down her throat."

"Oh, boy, just what we need—a scar on her neck! What's her mother going to think about that?"

"That's show business," Matt said. "I'd worry about the patient instead of her mother at this point."

The patient was wheeled into the operating room with anesthesia standing by. The area over the windpipe was infiltrated with local anesthetic. It was obvious that Dr. Gold was nervous. His hands were shaking and he had been drinking. A tube had been put through her mouth to suck out the stomach so she wouldn't aspirate. She was thrashing around even though she had been sedated.

"Do you want me to do it?"

"Would you?" asked Dr. Gold, as he handed Matt the scalpel.

He quickly made an incision over the windpipe, clamped the anterior veins beneath the skin and quickly tied them with silk. He cut down to the tracheal rings around the windpipe and put a hook into the upper tracheal ring with his left hand and made a sharp one-half inch cut in the windpipe. Past experience reminded him to duck his head as her cough reflex blew a mucous plug up to the ceiling. He quickly slipped the anesthesia tube in place and anchored it with silk. This was then hooked up to the anesthesia machine and the patient was put to sleep.

Dr. Gold then took down the elaborate dressing. The blood was oozing from the wound in several places. He used the cautery on bleeders he could see and then put a new anterior and posterior pack in the nose and tightened it down to create pressure in the back of the throat. The packing slowed the bleeding. The patient was sent back to the recovery room. It was almost 6:00 A.M. and Matt would soon be leaving the hospital.

"What should I do?" Dr. Gold asked.

"I think you ought to get a hematologist in to see her as an emergency. She doesn't seem to be clotting her blood very well. She's had enough new blood added so it may be screwing up her clotting mechanism. You've got a big problem here. Get all the help you can get."

Before Matt left the hospital to return uptown to Sloan, Annie stopped him in the foyer. "Dr. Kendall, Dr. Allen, the ophthalmologist, came in to see Mrs. Domkowski. He told her your judgment was right on the money. He took the foreign body out and told her she was lucky she didn't lose all the vision in her right eye. And he left an envelope for you in your box."

"Thanks, Annie."

Matt caught a bus on Lexington Avenue and opened the envelope.

There were two tickets for the new Broadway show "How to Succeed in Business Without Really Trying." He decided that all that work had been worth it. He and Nancy had wanted to see that show but they couldn't afford the tickets.

The following Friday, when he went back to work at Manhattan General, there was another envelope waiting for him. This time it was from Dr. Gold with $20 in it and a note. "Thanks a lot! The hematologist found out she had a blood defect (a factor five deficiency) and that's why she couldn't clot her blood. She was given the necessary blood replacements and promptly stopped bleeding."

Matt replaced the twenty in the envelope. He added a note: "Thanks but no thanks. Keep your money. And keep your thanks, too. That girl could have suffered less if you'd been accessible." Matt sealed the money and the note and put it in Gold's mail slot. He only hesitated once before turning and walking out the door of the hospital.

9

THE SURGICAL ONCOLOGY FELLOWSHIP at Memorial Sloan Kettering was one of the most sought-after fellowships in the country—six fellows were appointed each year.

Each service had an anatomical area for research and clinical study and treatment. They were all excellent—a few were outstanding. Matt had his favorites.

His first surgical rotation at Memorial Hospital was on the urology service. The chief of the service was a dynamic young urologist named Dr. Will Whitney. The first day he scrubbed with Dr. Whitney, he was really impressed. Dr. Whitney was a tall, good-looking man with a sagacious temperment and excellent surgical technique.

"I'm going to teach you how to do this operation so you'll be able to do it blindfolded," he told Matt.

"That's OK with me."

The next Monday, Dr. Whitney scheduled two patients for radical resections of bladders for cancer and the formation of ileal bladders to hold the urine. Each patient had invasive cancer of the bladder. The treatment was to surgically remove the bladder (cystectomy) if the tumor hadn't spread too far.

Dr. Whitney made a large incision in the midline of the lower abdomen. He used cloth pads to pack off the bowel. He then located the two tubes (ureters) that drain the kidneys and cut the distal ends. He cut out the entire urinary bladder and the lymph glands along the pelvic rim. A segment of distal small bowel was then isolated with its blood vessels and the cut ends of the ureters were implanted into it, creating an artificial bladder. One end of the small bowel was brought out to the skin surface for drainage. It was a real pleasure to watch Will work because he made it look easy. He had long, slender fingers and was meticulous in his dissection, handling the tissues ever so gently.

That next week, Dr. Whitney operated on five patients with bladder cancer. The delicate, methodical way he worked was like listening to the Vienna Symphony play Mozart. He was equally adept at all operations: kidney resections, cancers of the testicles, and prostates.

Whitney emphasized clamping the renal vein before doing kidney resections to prevent tumor emboli from going to the lungs. He did not want a piece of the kidney cancer to break off and travel.

"We've got a real difficult kidney case coming in next week," he told Matt. "It's a young lady. Order an inferior vena cavagram when she comes in and we'll work on it together."

A vena cavagram is an x-ray picture of the largest vein that goes from the kidney and liver to the heart. The study is usually done by placing a sterile plastic tube in a vein in the leg and directing the tube to the area around the kidney. A bolus of dye is injected into the tube, and x-ray pictures are taken that show what's going on within the blood vessels.

Matt and Dr. Whitney looked at the x-rays together with the radiologist.

"It looks like that kidney tumor is growing into that large vein," said Matt. "It's just waiting to break off and spread to the lungs."

"That's right," said Dr. Whitney. "This operation could be a real challenge. We're going to take that tumor out before it breaks off. Order a few extra units of blood. Get a good night's sleep Thursday night. We'll be doing the case on Friday."

In the OR on Friday, Whitney made a large flank incision and most of the surgical dissection was done to clear the area around the kidney and the vena cava. Vascular loops were put above and below the large vein that went to the heart, in case too much blood was lost.

A small incision was made in the renal vein and vena cava, and as the blood leaked out and flowed, Whitney, using long, fine metal pickups, removed the tumor thrombus. A heavy tie was then placed around the kidney vein.

While Whitney was working and the blood was leaking out of the vein, Matt used a large metal sucker to suck the blood out of the wound so that he could see where to suture the hole. The cancerous kidney was then removed. It was a slick job.

"That worked great!" said Matt.

"Only time will tell if she gets any tumor emboli into her lungs," remarked Whitney.

* * *

Matt's next rotation was on the breast service. There were eight attending surgeons with varying degrees of expertise. The volume of surgery was tremendous, although Dr. Fred Dare did most of it.

Sticking a needle into a suspicious breast lump was in vogue and was done the night before surgery by the residents to expedite the tumor diagnosis. The microscopic slides were often read by Dr. Ross prior to surgery.

Radical mastectomy was the treatment of choice for most breast cancers. However, in some medial quadrant tumors an ultra radical chest wall resection was done. Patients who had metastatic breast cancer, usually involving bone, were often treated by removing the ovaries or adrenal glands or both. These glands are the main sources of estrogen hormones and by removing them, hopefully, slow down the growth of the breast cancer.

Fred Dare did six or eight breast biopsies a day and sometimes two or three radical mastectomies. The breast lump was biopsied; a frozen section tissue diagnosis was made, and if it was cancer, a radical mastectomy was performed.

Matt was helping Dr. Dare do a breast biopsy on a 34-year-old nurse. She was listed on the schedule for a right breast biopsy. Dr. Dare would often check both breasts before proceeding with the biopsy. He felt a lump in the left breast.

"I think the left breast has more trouble than the right," said Dare. "Take a feel, Matt, see what you think."

"It feels like it has a bigger lump than the right," replied Matt.

Dr. Dare did the biopsy on the left and it came back cancer. So he proceeded to do a left radical mastectomy.

The next day when the patient was fully awake, she was angry and perplexed. She panicked. Matt was called to see her.

"Dr. Dare took the wrong breast off!" she screamed with tears coming down her cheeks.

Matt tried to explain to her what had happened.

"Dr. Dare examined your breasts while you were asleep and thought your left breast had more trouble than your right."

"I don't believe it!" she hollered.

"It's the truth," said Matt.

"I can't accept that!" said the patient. "He told me my right breast was going to be biopsied!"

"Calm down. I'll call Dr. Dare and have him explain what happened."

Matt called Dr. Dare's office and told him about the nurse. He said he'd be over after his office hours. Matt was to meet him on the floor.

At 5:30 the two walked into the patient's room. Before the patient could say anything, Dr. Dare spoke up. "Young lady, the gods must be keeping an eye on you. I was going to biopsy your right breast but instead I did your left breast. We took the cancer out that could destroy your life! If we had biopsied your right breast and ignored the left, that cancer would have kept growing without anyone knowing about it."

"But what about the tumor in my right breast?" she asked.

"We'll biopsy that one in a few days. I'm sure it's nothing," said Dr. Dare. "Matt, schedule her for a biopsy in a couple of days."

A few days later, it was biopsied.

Fortunately, it was nothing and the patient left the hospital happy. No malpractice suit was instituted.

The following week, Matt was scheduled to help a young attending surgeon do a bilateral adrenalectomy on a breast cancer patient with metastatic cancer. The patient's bones were riddled with cancer. He had scrubbed on a few adrenalectomies at Whitestone Hospital and was looking forward to seeing how they did the operation at Sloan.

The adrenal glands are two small fan-shaped glands that sit on the upper poles of the kidneys under the diaphragm and sometimes can be difficult to find and are not easy to remove. The right gland is the most difficult to resect because it is under the liver and close to the major blood vessels that return the blood to the heart. The left is easier.

The young attending, Dr. John Allen, made a large flank incision on the right side and located the kidney. He did some sharp dissection and finally visualized what appeared to be the right adrenal gland. The operative field was quite bloody and Matt was using the suction apparatus frequently to suck out the blood.

"I wonder where the hell that central vein is," said Dr. Allen. "The one that goes to the vena cava. It's a bugger to find."

"Why don't we tie up some of these bleeders and irrigate the wound first?" suggested Matt. "We'll be able to see better. We don't want to tear off that vein."

"You're right," said Allen.

They finally found the short vein and tied it off. After they completed the right side, the patient was turned on the operating table for the left side.

"Matt, why don't you let the junior resident, Dr. Rashid, help me on the left side. You hold the retractors so he can learn how to do it."

"OK!" replied Matt.

Ronish Rashid had his surgical boards from the Royal College of Surgeons in England and was an accomplished surgeon. He was beginning his residency at Sloan. It was obvious that Dr. Allen was trying to impress him.

After making the flank incision on the left side and doing some dissecting he remarked, "Dr. Rashid, we're approaching the left adrenal gland. It looks like it's a big one."

"I think you're too low in your dissection," Rashid replied.

"Not really," Allen said, as he proceeded to clip the blood vessels around the gland. "This is a good-sized one for you to see."

"Why don't you show it to Matt?" said Dr. Rashid.

"OK. Exchange places."

When Matt saw what was going on he realized why Dr. Rashid had suggested the switch.

"I think you're dissecting out the tail of the pancreas," said Matt to the attending. "The adrenal's tucked up higher."

"Huh? Are you sure?"

"Yes. I'm sure," said Matt.

The attending changed his approach and finally found the left adrenal tucked under the diaphragm.

"We'd better drain this left side well in case there's a problem," suggested Matt.

The following week the patient almost died. She sloughed the tail of her pancreas and developed a pancreatitis and a draining pancreatic fistula.

When Dr. Allen clipped all those blood vessels around the tail of the pancreas, it became necrotic because there were no nutrients going to it. She was hospitalized for over a month but finally recovered.

Matt's next rotation was on the gastric and mixed tumor service during the time when the James Ewing Society had its annual scientific meeting in New York City.

Leading cancer specialists from all over the world came to the Memorial Cancer Center to present research papers and to discuss new methods of treatment.

While that meeting was in session, most of the surgical chiefs scheduled unusual, difficult operations so they could impress the visiting doctors. Surgeons from England, Europe, and the Far East were often in the audience.

Matt was scheduled to assist Dr. George Packard, along with a junior resident, in the resection of a right lobe of a liver for cancer. Dr. Packard was the chief of the gastric and mixed tumor service and was an internationally known surgeon who had operated on Eva Peron and a number of other famous people.

Resection of the right lobe of the liver had been attempted many times before. Too often, the results were tragic and frequently the patient would die, either in the operating room from hemorrhage, or from complications during the 30 days following surgery.

Dr. Packard had selected the liver resection case for the audience to demonstrate his operating expertise. He was by far the best technical surgeon that Matt had ever seen. He seemed ambidextrous—able to use both hands for clamping, suturing or dissection. The scrub nurses, who enjoyed a challenge, were always eager to scrub for him.

The patient he was going to operate on was the mother of the chief of surgery at one of the university centers in Ohio. She was 63 years old and had had a colon resection done four years before. She now presented with an enlarged right lobe of her liver. A needle biopsy of the liver confirmed that she had a metastatic cancer in the right lobe.

The professor had accompanied his mother to New York for the surgical procedure. The patient's heart and lungs were in good shape, although she was slightly anemic. A barium enema had been done to see if she had any recurrent tumor in the bowel. As far as could be determined the only tumor present was in the right lobe of her liver. The patient was thin, weighing 120 pounds, and was a good candidate for Dr. Packard to demonstrate his surgical prowess.

The case was scheduled for 8:30 A.M. in the main amphitheater of the operating room. The area surrounding the operating room was packed with visiting surgeons before Dr. Packard's arrival.

Matt presented the case to the assembled doctors. The anesthesiologist put the patient to sleep and the patient was prepped with an antiseptic solution. Sterile drapes were placed around the operating field.

Dr. Packard made his dramatic appearance. He was a relatively short, stocky man with alert, keen eyes. He had been a successful pathologist at Yale Medical School before deciding to become a cancer surgeon and his self assurance was quite noticeable.

"Gentlemen, I plan to make a large T-shaped incision over the right upper abdomen and extend it into the chest to expose the liver and the vena cava. As you know, the vena cava is the main venous conduit for return of the blood to the heart. We'll enter the chest and put a tape around the upper part of that vessel that goes through the liver and place a tape on the vessel below the liver in the abdomen. This will help control any bleeding that may occur.

"Since the liver has a blood supply that goes to each lobe and a bile drainage system from each lobe, we'll isolate those structures and tie them off first. We'll be doing a right liver resection and, therefore, we'll take the gallbladder out also.

"The most dangerous part of the operation is to suture ligate the many small hepatic veins that empty into the vena cava, on the undersurface of the liver. If you miss one of those, it can be fatal."

Just as he said that, Dr. Packard told Matt to release a clamp on a small hepatic vein. The clamp snapped off too early and the blood started to well up underneath the liver. Packard quickly grabbed an arterial suture and whipstitched the area. The tie was placed, and with the blood filling up the wound, he tied the suture perfectly. Matt then used suction to clean out the blood. Packard quickly completed the resection of the right lobe.

"I didn't mean to demonstrate what you shouldn't do," said Packard. "But if you're lucky, like I just was, the patient will survive." In a soft voice, Dr. Packard said, "Drop that lousy clamp off the field, Matt."

As if it had been the end of a symphony, the audience stood up and applauded. The surgeons in the audience shook their heads in amazement. Only three units of blood were necessary to replace the blood lost during the entire liver resection. Drains were put in place and Dr. Packard helped the two residents start the wound closure.

"Matt, I want the two of you to come up to the locker room to meet this woman's son, the professor from Ohio. I'll be talking to the visiting surgeons there."

When the residents finished closing the wound, they went up to the locker room while Dr. Packard was taking a shower. The professor was sitting on a sofa looking at the East River skyline.

"I want to thank you for assisting Dr. Packard do the operation on my mother."

"You're very welcome, Sir," responded Matt.

"I used to think I was God when I operated back in Ohio. I now know I'm not. I just saw God operate. George is a magnificent surgeon."

"He's the greatest," said the residents.

When Packard finished his shower and dressed, he came out.

"Have you boys met the professor?"

"We just had the pleasure."

"Keep a close eye on his mother tonight."

The crème de la crème of surgical training at Memorial Sloan Kettering Cancer Center was the head and neck service. Each surgical fellow rotated through this service during the last six months of training. Dr. Edgar Hayes, known as the Father of Head and Neck Surgery, was the chief of the service and had championed the radical surgical approach for head and neck cancer. He was internationally known and had assembled some of the top head and neck surgeons in the country to join his service. Each, under his tutelage, was assigned a sub-specialty in the head and neck area to assess and develop new techniques and treatments.

Head and neck weekly morbidity and mortality conferences were held and new patients were presented to Dr. Hayes by the resident surgeons-in-training. Opinions as to the best treatment for each patient were discussed. Every major complication and death would be reviewed. The audience was filled with visiting doctors from around the world. Dr. Hayes made the final judgment on each case, upon completion of a consensus of the attending surgeons.

The volume of head and neck surgery at Sloan was incredible. Patients arrived from all over the world for treatment: combined monoblock resections of the mandible and glands in the neck, parotid resections, maxilla resections, laryngectomies, and thyroid resections were done daily. The chief surgical resident on the head and neck service saw the whole gamut of old and new surgical procedures.

Most of the surgery done on the head and neck service by the attending staff was excellent. Because there were residents in training doing surgery, accidents happened that were life-threatening to some of the patients.

On rare occasions, a child developed cancer and this is most traumatic for the child and for the surgeon who has to operate.

Matt would never forget a particular case in a child that he saw on service when he was one of the chief resident surgeons.

A five-year-old child was admitted to the head and neck service with a large facial maxillary sinus cancer, pushing the cheek forward with a bulging mass and obstructing the posterior throat, causing breathing problems.

A preliminary tracheostomy, (an opening in the neck) had to be done before anesthesia could be administered for the surgery. In other words, an airway through a tube in the neck would be established prior to the surgery because the tumor obstructed the upper airway in the mouth.

The chief surgical resident was to do the tracheostomy, and then an attending head and neck surgeon would help in the difficult radical sinus surgery.

Establishing an airway in a child is a much more difficult procedure than in an adult, because the anatomical structures are so much smaller and difficult to delineate. In an adult, the larynx and bronchus that goes to the lungs form a larger round opening and it's easier to insert a metal tracheostomy tube.

Intravenous tubing for fluids and medication is first put in the child's arm for sedation. A local anesthetic is injected through a needle in the neck area over the trachea and the chief resident surgeon then made an incision.

The small veins that were encountered were clamped and tied and the procedure seemed to be going well. A scalpel cut was made in the cartilaginous ring of the main bronchus to the lungs so that a metal tube could be inserted. The child started to cough and struggle. The chief surgical resident had difficulty getting the metal tracheostomy tube into the opening in the airway. With a hard push, he announced: "I've got the trach tube in."

The anesthesiologist attempted to hook up pure oxygen to the end of the metal trach tube, but the child continued to struggle.

"Try to listen to the lungs to see if the air is getting in," the anesthesiologist called out. A stethescope was placed over the child's lungs.

"I don't hear any air getting through," said his assistant.

"I don't think that trach is in the right place," said the senior anesthesiologist. "You're going to have to replace it."

"That tube is in the right place!" shouted the resident.

The chief resident surgeon tried to suction out the tube by placing a long rubber tube down the opening. It didn't go down. The child got worse. Soon the child was no longer struggling and was placid. There was still a heartbeat and rapid pulse.

One of the attending head and neck surgeons who had been scrubbing came into the operating room. "What's wrong here?" he asked.

"We're losing her!" replied the anesthesiologist. "She's not aerating."

The attending surgeon shoved the senior resident out of the way, pulled the trach tube out, and told the resident to push on the child's chest. A bloody plug was coughed up. He held the trach open with a clamp and sucked out the mucous and blood.

"We've got a real problem here," he said. "You shoved that trach tube through the posterior wall of the trachea into the esophagus. No wonder she can't breathe." He gently put the trach tube into the proper place in the airway and said, "We're going to have to explore this neck and close the tear in the esophagus behind the trach. How's she doing?"

"OK, so far."

"Give her some intravenous antibiotics," he said.

He quickly made a larger incision in the neck and sharply dissected down to the tear in the esophagus. There was some bleeding in the tissues that helped identify the perforation made by the metal tube.

The small hole was quickly sutured with silk and suction drains were placed next to the area to keep it clear.

"That's all we can do today," said the head and neck attending surgeon. "When she gets better we'll resect that sinus tumor."

Eventually the chief resident on the head and neck service operated with Dr. Edgar Hayes. This was quite an experience. Dr. Hayes worked in the afternoon from 1:00 to 5:00 in one of the main amphitheater operating rooms. Matt's first encounter with Dr. Hayes was awesome. He had booked three parotid tumor cases to do in one afternoon.

Back home at Whitestone Hospital, one parotid tumor case would be booked for five hours. Here at Sloan, Hayes had booked three cases to do in the same timeframe. Matt couldn't believe it. He had thought he'd be in the operating room until midnight.

The first case was a 56-year-old white male, who had been operated on in upstate New York for a large parotid tumor in front of his left ear. The tumor was the size of a hen's egg and the surgeon in upstate New York had trouble with bleeding and was unsure of the location of the facial nerve that controls the muscles of the face, the eye and the lip. He backed out of the operation. That surgeon felt that retreat was the better part of valor. There was a fresh scar in front of the patient's ear.

The anesthesiologist passed an endotracheal tube down the patient's throat and Matt prepped the area and draped the face and neck before Dr. Hayes entered the operating room. Dr. Hayes was a tall man and the operating table was adjusted to his height. Matt took his place opposite him to assist in the operation.

Hayes quickly made a sharp incision in front of the ear and developed skin flaps to expose the salivary gland tumor. He then placed his stubby forefinger against the ear canal and said to Matt, "The main trunk of the facial nerve is usually right here. Watch closely."

Using sharp-pointed scissors he spread and cut the gland in front of the facial nerve. It took him ten minutes to identify it. There was a brisk bleeder clouding the field so Matt made a quick pass at the bleeder with a clamp.

Hayes gently pushed his hand away. "If anyone's going to clamp the facial nerve, I'd like that privilege. Use the suction!"

Hayes continued to cut and dissect around the tumor as Matt used the metal sucker to drain the blood. He then gave Matt a special sterile soup spoon to use to help retract the tumor—it actually looked like a real soup spoon.

It took Dr. Hayes about 30 minutes to remove the tumor. He then clamped the bleeders and placed a drain in the wound. Matt closed the skin and applied the wound dressing.

That afternoon Dr. Hayes did two more cases and was through operating by 5:00 P.M.

The following Friday, Matt was on call for admission work-ups on the head and neck service. Dr. Hayes spoke to him about a prominent female movie star who was being admitted.

"Matt, a movie star will be arriving from London later this afternoon. I plan to remove a small skin cancer from her upper lip area in the operating room Saturday morning. Sir Stafford Blade, a prominent British surgeon, saw her in London. He called me and he thinks she might have a melanoma. You're to treat her like any other patient and don't let her pull any nonsense."

"Is she likely to?"

"He told me that she became hysterical when he told her about the possibility of a melanoma. Celebrities can be demanding."

Around 7 P.M. Matt received a call from the head nurse on one of the floors on the Gold Coast, where the patients had their own private baths. "Dr. Kendall, we have a problem up here," said Sara Morse, the head nurse. "Joan Garnett, the movie star, is here with seventeen pieces of luggage and she insists on keeping all of it with her in her room. Her luggage is filling up the entire hallway. Her husband is with her and he's some big movie mogul insisting that she needs a bigger room."

"Well, give her a bigger room."

"She's got the biggest end room now," said the head nurse. "The room won't hold seventeen pieces of luggage and the bed."

"Well, tell her if she wants a place to sleep, she'll have to get rid of some of her luggage."

"You tell her," said the nurse.

Matt thought about it for a minute. "Tell her she can pick out any three pieces of luggage and the rest will have to be put in storage."

"You come up here and tell her that."

"OK, I'll be right up," replied Matt. After all, Edgar Hayes told him to expect anything and he was to treat her like any other patient.

When he saw Joan Garnett, she looked beautiful—from a distance. When he got close it was obvious she had a professional makeup job.

She looked Matt straight in the eye and said, "Who are you to tell me that I can only have three pieces of luggage?"

"I'm one of the doctors on the head and neck service and I'll be examining you prior to your surgery."

"I'm not going to have any intern examining me."

"I'm not an intern. I'm the chief surgical resident on Dr. Hayes' service, and will be helping him do your surgery."

"You look awfully young to be doing surgery."

"Thank you," he replied.

"Well, I'm still not going to let you examine me."

"Then you'll have to leave. Dr. Hayes will not do your surgery unless you have a physical exam, chest x-ray, electrocardiogram, and some blood work."

"Ugh. You mean they'll put a needle in my arm?"

"That's right."

"Well, that does it! I'm leaving! I'm not going to let a young whippersnapper like you tell *me* what to do!"

"Mrs. Garnett," said Matt as calmly as he could, "you happen to be in the largest and best cancer hospital in the world. Dr. Hayes is the best head and neck surgeon in the world. It's your choice, if you choose to leave. That prominent British surgeon didn't send you here to complain about your luggage and physical exam."

She grabbed her husband's arm, stormed down the hall, and took the elevator to the lobby.

"Joan, wait! You'd better reconsider," advised her husband.

"I'm going to call Dr. Shepard, my psychiatrist on Park Avenue."

She made the call and was instructed to go back to her room and to let Dr. Kendall examine her.

She reluctantly went back to her room, picked out three suitcases and said, "I guess I have to let you examine me. I'd prefer that you come back in a half hour so I can fix my makeup and get settled."

"I'll do that," replied Matt. "There's something else I have to tell you. You'll have to remove your makeup from the area above your lip where the black mole is."

"My God," she yelled. "I might as well take my clothes off if I need to take my makeup off!"

"That's the other thing," said Matt. "You'll have to disrobe for my examination."

"What's next?"

He continued to make his nightly rounds on the wards, seeing the sick patients and writing orders that were needed. He finally got a call from the head nurse stating that Joan Garnett was ready, so he took an elevator to the floor. When he got to her room, she was lying on the bed with an expensive-looking negligee and bed jacket on.

Matt did his routine eye, ear, nose, and throat exam and had difficulty seeing the small black mole over her left upper lip. He listened to her heart and lungs and noticed that she had full upper body cosmetics on. It was the first time he had seen someone with makeup over their chest and neck area. He took her blood pressure and pulse and examined her abdomen, which was flat and athletic. He did a brief neurological exam to check her reflexes, which were all normal. While doing the examination, he took a complete history concerning sun exposure, the time the mole was first noticed, and made notes of any pertinent history.

The next morning he made head and neck rounds on the sick patients with Dr. Hayes and the rest of the resident staff. "Matt, I understand that movie star gave you a hard time last night. Miss Morse on the Phipps Pavilion told me about it."

"I've handled tougher."

"I understand she threatened to leave the hospital and refused to let you do a physical exam?"

"At first she refused, but she eventually let me examine her."

When they got to the scrub room to wash their hands, Dr. Hayes persisted about finding out what had transpired the night before. "Do you think she has a melanoma?"

"No, I don't think so. But I haven't seen very many skin melanomas."

"Well, when you see one, you'll recognize it."

When they got into the operating room, there was silence. The movie star had no makeup on whatsoever and she looked quite a bit older. Matt prepared the area to be excised with an antiseptic soap solution and drapes were placed around her head. Intravenous medication had been given to sedate her. Then a syringe with local anesthesia was used to anesthetize the area over her lip.

The scrub nurse handed the scalpel to Dr. Hayes and he quickly and deftly excised the mole. Using fine suture material he quickly closed the wound. The operation took ten minutes. The tissue was given to the pathologist, who stated the diagnosis could not be established until permanent tissue sections were done. However, he felt it would be benign. By the time the drapes were removed the patient was wide awake.

Dr. Hayes spoke up, "It looks like you don't have a cancer. We'll know definitely in a few days. There is something I want to talk to you about, though. I believe you owe this young doctor assisting me an apology for the way you acted last night. I'd like to hear it from you."

The movie star got red as a beet. She hesitated and then said, "I'm sorry, young man. I did act a little immature. I guess I was feeling the pressure."

"We are all under pressure here, Miss Garnett—all of us," said Dr. Hayes. He turned around and walked out of the operating room.

That was not the end of it. One week later a large box was delivered to Matt's apartment. When he got home from work he opened it to find six bottles of expensive Dom Perignon French champagne. There was a card in the box, signed simply, "Joan." The address of the liquor store it came from was also on the box.

The next day, Matt went to the store and told the owner his wife didn't like champagne. The proprietor told him that each of those six bottles was good as gold. It was one of their most expensive champagnes.

"How would you like to take it all back and let me establish a credit line?"

"That's fine with me, young man. I can always sell that champagne!"

He went home and wrote a card to Joan Garnett in care of the Hollywood studio. "Mrs. Garnett," it read, "Thanks for the bubbly, and good luck to you. I'm glad your tumor was benign."

10

BEFORE MATT COMPLETED his surgical fellowship in New York City, he was offered the opportunity to stay on the attending staff at Memorial Sloan Kettering Hospital.

He and his wife had discussed the advantages and disadvantages of staying in New York City. Nancy did not like New York, to put it mildly, and thought it would be the wrong place to bring up children.

The following week, a major calamity occurred that had a profound influence on their decision. Matt was working in the operating room, assisting Dr. Hayes on a head and neck case, when the operating supervisor came into the room.

"Dr. Hayes, I'd like to interrupt. Dr. Kendall has an urgent message."

"Go right ahead. It's all right," said Hayes, as he stopped operating.

"Dr. Kendall, your wife is in the Metropolitan Hospital Emergency Room. Evidently, she was attacked in Central Park. She seems to be OK except for an arm injury. The emergency room nurse said to tell you that your two children are not injured. They're x-raying your wife's arm. She may have a fracture."

"Get me another resident immediately," said Dr. Hayes. Matt, you'd better go see what's going on. Let me know if you need any help. Keep my office posted."

"Thanks!" replied Matt.

Another surgical resident came in to replace him. He quickly dressed in his street clothes and took a cab to Metropolitan Hospital. When he got to the emergency room he could hear two children screaming at the top of their lungs and all he had to do was follow the noise to find them. His wife was being x-rayed in the x-ray department and seen by an orthopedic doctor.

The children stopped crying when they saw their father. He picked up Mike and gave Betsy a hug.

"I'd like to talk to whoever is taking care of my wife," he said, "I'm a surgical resident over at Sloan Kettering."

"I'll get one of the doctors to talk to you," replied the ER nurse.

Dr. Stetson, an orthopedic resident, came into the waiting room area. "There's some good news. Your wife does not have a fracture. However, she has a large hematoma in her upper arm and some muscle damage. You'll have to pack her arm in ice intermittently today."

"We'll do whatever you think is best. What happened?"

"Your wife was struck on her left upper arm with a broom handle as she was pushing the stroller. According to her, her pocketbook fell to the ground and a young boy grabbed the pocketbook. The attacker and the boy disappeared in the trees in Central Park. An elderly gentleman walking in the park saw the whole thing and ran over and helped her up and watched the kids. A policeman on horseback arrived and a police cruiser was called. Your wife and your children were brought here."

Fortunately, she did not have a fracture and was discharged. Matt stayed at home to take care of his wife for a few days. During that time, they talked. "I'm not going to stay in New York City," said Nancy. "I don't think that I would survive. It's lucky our kids weren't killed."

They finally decided to go back to New England. Matt would apply for surgical privileges at Whitestone Hospital.

Obtaining surgical privileges at a big city hospital is not easy. It can be a political hassle, no matter how good your training background. Adding a new surgeon to a staff creates anxieties for the other surgeons because there is someone else competing for a piece of the pie. When Matt returned to the hospital he had trained at, he followed protocol and arranged to meet with the Chief of Surgery, Dr. Philip McBratney.

"Good to see you, Matt. I got your letter from New York and think it's a good idea we talk. I also received letters from your chiefs of surgery at Sloan Kettering Cancer Center. Your recommendations are excellent. I will add, however, that you are creating some anxiety among the younger surgeons here who do not have your training background. They want you to define just what you plan to do, and so do I. Let's hear it."

"I'm primarily interested in doing tumor surgery. I want to be a surgical oncologist."

"Well, you're not in New York City any more," said Dr. McBratney. "The population base here is nothing like it is there. I'm not sure we can support two cancer specialists and still keep the general surgeons happy. The general surgeons like to do tumor surgery also. Dr. Bob Walker, our other cancer surgeon, is less than delighted about your coming back."

"With my three and a half years of additional surgical training in New York, I think I can add some new expertise to the staff, particularly on the difficult tumor cases. We both know Dr. Walker is getting old—besides, there are some new surgical techniques now being used in the treatment of cancer in New York City."

"Well, I have to tell you, we had a close vote in our surgical staff meeting. Dr. Walker disapproved of giving you privileges. He gave a dramatic, impassioned talk about your threat."

"I might have done the same if I were in his shoes."

"There's no way, with your background, we can keep you out," said Dr. McBratney. However, you're going to have a tough row to hoe. We voted to restrict your surgical privileges to tumor cases. You won't be able to do the bread and butter surgery of the general surgeons; hernias, gallbladders, hemorrhoids, etcetera. The surgical staff also voted not to let you work in the emergency room seeing unassigned cases."

"That's unfair!" said Matt. "That's how you get started, working in the ER."

"I know," said McBratney. "Most of our general surgeons get started that way. That's how they get their name known to the general practitioners and internists who see the patients first."

"I see the general surgeons are giving me a big welcome and homecoming. Economics come first!"

"That's right," said McBratney. "You're now out in the real world. If you're any good, you'll succeed. If you're a run-of-the-mill surgeon, you won't survive. But if you've got a gift, you might just make a contribution to our staff. There also are some other requirements that you must fulfill before you can start doing surgery at this hospital. You have to get an office to practice in before getting hospital admitting privileges."

"How am I supposed to do that?" Matt asked.

"You'll have to work that out on your own."

This certainly wasn't what he had anticipated. The *old boys* controlled the hospital. It was worse than the obstacle course he had to pass when he was a navy air corps cadet. He talked to his older brother, who was a lawyer, about borrowing some money to start his practice.

His brother came through, and Matt moved into an old house in an outlying town, about 15 miles west of the capital. He and his wife and two children lived in the upstairs of the building, and he borrowed money for an old desk, examining table, and an overhead surgical light. After renovating a couple of rooms downstairs he scraped together enough money to get a sterilizer and a few surgical instruments so he could sew up lacerations and do a few skin and tissue biopsies. It would be his own little E.R. in his home. It would help him pay the rent.

Nancy was helpful because she could act as a secretary and a nurse when he saw his patients. One problem developed when he started practice in that old house. He had two little children running around and their curiosity would occasionally interrupt the decorum, particularly if someone knocked on the door with a youngster who had a laceration that needed to be stitched. Trying to hold down a child while you suture a laceration can be quite frustrating, especially when your own child is curious about the procedure.

One day, Betsy, who was five years old, walked into the examining room when stitches were being applied.

"She's got a big boo-boo, hasn't she?"

"Yes, Betsy. Now go back into the living room," said her dad.

"I want to watch," said Betsy. "She's bleeding."

"I know. Be a nice girl and go back into the living room and watch TV."

"I'm staying," she said.

"You don't want a spanking, do you?"

"No," said Betsy as she stuck out her lower lip and stomped out of the room.

Three months after Matt started his surgical practice, Dr. Stronghart, the Chief of Urology, whom Matt had assisted on his first surgical operation at Whitestone Hospital, stopped him in the hallway.

"Matt, I hear some of the senior general surgical *old boys* are trying to give you the business."

"That's right."

"Well I don't like it! I never did like Bob Walker! He's a pompous ass and a loner. They're afraid of a little healthy competition! I'm inviting you to come and use my office in the medical building so you can get started. You won't be busy in the beginning so my secretary can take your calls, if you'll pay for your own phone."

"Thanks a lot," said Matt. "I'll do it. That's great!"

Matt called the phone company and he moved in the next day. He now had a base next to the hospital in which to see his patients. He was beginning to break down the political barrier.

Dr. Stronghart talked to some of his colleagues. Soon, colon cancer cases were being referred to Matt's office. Many times the urologists would do barium enema studies of the rectum and colon on their prostatic cancer cases and if they found a colon cancer, Matt would be called in.

The chief of the ear, nose and throat service started to refer a few head and neck cancer cases to him and soon he started doing major resections of oral cancers and extensive radical neck dissections. Word got around that he could do a good neck dissection. He started to give Bob Walker competition. His training in New York was beginning to pay off.

The small outlying community that Matt lived in began to play an increasing part in the development of his surgical practice. The townspeople soon realized that he knew a lot about bellyaches and tumors. He was always available because he kept his home and office in the same building. People would drive up at any time of day or night and knock on the door for help. Some of these small cases helped pay the rent and later led to bigger surgical cases.

There was also a change in the hierarchy of the surgical staff. Dr. Stanley had retired, Dr. McBratney had died, and there was a new young chief of surgery, Dr. Jack Diamond.

As Matt continued his surgical practice, he still maintained an office in his home. On a Sunday morning, while the family was eating breakfast, there was a knock on the back door. He opened the door and there was a lady with a small boy standing in front of her. She spoke in broken English. "My boy is sick," she said. "He told me to take him to the doctor."

"What happened?" asked Matt as he looked at the boy, who appeared quite pale. The boy spoke up.

"I went sledding this morning and it was icy. I rolled off the side of my sled and hit a tree. There's something broken inside."

Matt quickly examined him. He was exquisitely tender in the left upper abdomen and chest area. He flinched when he pressed on his sternum and his pulse was rapid. "Call the hospital emergency room," he said to Nancy. "Tell them I'm bringing in a youngster with a possible ruptured spleen. Call Dr. Mack, the chief resident, and have him meet me there."

He put the boy and his mother into his car and drove as fast as he could to the hospital. The little boy looked deathly sick and was diaphoretic and pale. The chief resident met them at the door. "Whatcha got?" asked Dr. Mack.

"Possible ruptured spleen," said Matt. "Get an intravenous line into him for fluid replacement and have them type and cross-match three units of blood as fast as they can. Do a stat hematocrit to see how much blood he's lost." A quick x-ray of the abdomen was taken, suggesting a ruptured spleen, and the boy was taken to the operating room.

The seven-year-old boy was quickly put to sleep and Matt made a liberal vertical incision in the left upper abdomen. When the abdomen was entered it was full of bright red blood with clots and a gush of blood spurted out. He scooped the clots out with his hands.

"You better pump the blood into him," said Matt to the anesthesiologist. "He looks like he's lost quite a bit. Pull harder on that retractor," he snapped at the intern.

Matt grabbed the spleen in his left hand and deftly cut the lateral ligaments between the left kidney and the spleen. He didn't have time to do a nice clean dissection and tie off the splenic artery. The boy was bleeding out, and his belly was filling up with blood. The boy's blood pressure was dropping. When Matt made sure of where he was, he took a large Kelly clamp and placed it across the splenic pedicle, where the blood vessels are that go to the spleen. It was a rough, rapid Bulgarian approach but it worked. Quickly they suctioned out the blood around the area and took the time to make sure the clamp was in the right place.

The anesthesiologist pumped blood into his veins to get his blood pressure back up, and once his pressure stabilized they proceeded to remove the spleen. Heavy silk suture ligatures were used to tie off the main blood vessels to the spleen and it was removed. The abdominal wound was quickly sewed up. The next day the boy was up and around as though nothing had happened to him. He had a smile on his face.

"I knew there was something broken in there," he told Matt.

"You were right, son. That man upstairs was keeping an eye on you."

As Matt's surgical practice expanded, more patients were in-service patients in the hospital. This meant he had to make rounds on a daily basis on these patients and see that they were getting better. The sick patients would have to be seen at least twice a day, more if needed. On weekends, there weren't as many doctors around the hospital, but he would still see his patients and walk through the wards.

He would occasionally meet general practitioners and internists and idle conversation often led to referrals for his practice. On occasion, he would be asked to comment or see one of their medical patients.

One Sunday, as he was seeing one of his Gold Coast patients, he walked out of his patient's room and an internist was waiting for him at the nursing station.

"Dr. Kendall, I'm Dr. Potwin. I've got a diagnostic problem that I'd like you to see for me. He's a fifty-four-year-old white-collar worker, who's an officer in one of our factories nearby and was helping a friend move a locker when he hurt his back."

"I'll be glad to see him," he said. "But maybe you need a bone specialist."

"No, it's not his back that bothers me, it's his belly. He's been in bed for four days. He doesn't want to get up and he's got abdominal distention. He's blown up like a balloon."

Matt went in to see him and decided to ask him some questions. "What happened to you, Mr. Black?"

"I was helping one of my employees move a locker. As we were moving it, I suddenly got this stabbing pain in my back and had to let go of the locker."

Sounds like an acute disc, thought Matt, but it's better to let the patient talk.

"The locker fell and I couldn't get up."

"Why?"

"Because the locker fell on top of me and they had to get two other guys to pull it off."

The man didn't look well. He was pale.

"Has he had a flat plate of the abdomen?"

"No," said Dr. Potwin. "I thought he might have had a coronary because he had chest pain when the locker fell on him. But the EKG was normal."

Matt stepped closer to the man and compressed the chest over the sternum with his fist.

"Ow! That hurts!" said the patient.

"Where?"

"On my ribs," he replied, as he placed his hand over his left chest.

Matt listened to his left chest. He could hear a slight rub.

"He needs chest and rib x-rays, stat. How's his blood work?"

"It was normal when he came in. He's been here four days," said Dr. Potwin.

Matt ordered the blood work and x-rays of the chest, ribs, and abdomen. Fortunately there was a good resident radiologist in the hospital who looked at the x-ray films.

"Your patient has four fractured ribs on the left side and his spleen shadow is enlarged," he reported.

More blood was drawn, including a type and cross-match in case blood was needed. Sure enough, the red cell count was down. The patient was taken to the operating room that Sunday afternoon and a ruptured spleen was found. There were two units of free-floating blood in the abdomen.

Matt decided to use a more classic approach in removing this spleen. He tied off the splenic artery first and then the short gastric arteries that went from the stomach to the spleen. He dissected the ligaments that attach to the spleen and gently removed it. It was a neater dissection. The next day, the patient's backache quickly disappeared.

The internist who asked him to see the patient was impressed. Dr. Kendall had another referring doctor.

11

IT WAS INEVITABLE that Matt would get involved with medical politics at Whitestone Hospital. He was specializing in cancer, a controversial field whose diagnostic methods and treatment were constantly changing. In order to play a role in those changes he would have to join or oppose the medical establishment. Even in his field of radical cancer surgery he started to realize that there had to be a better way to treat cancer. Radiation methods were improving and new drugs were being introduced. Doctors were beginning to specialize more frequently in medical oncology.

The opportunity to join or oppose the medical establishment came all too soon.

Matt had attended a meeting in Chicago of the American College of Surgeons and had heard and read about a new diagnostic method to detect breast cancer. It sounded promising so he decided to discuss the new technique with one of the younger radiologists, Dr. Paul Hooper.

Dr. Hooper was enthusiastic about the new method, since he had read about the technique developed by Dr. Egan who had trained at the M.D. Anderson Hospital in Houston, Texas. It was an x-ray method of imaging the breast, called mammography. It was introduced in 1913 in Germany by a surgeon named Solomon and was thought to be primitive, hazardous, and a curiosity. It didn't get medical support at that time.

In 1960 Egan published his experience with 1,000 breast cases and with the publication of his report there was a renewed interest in mammography.

Matt and Dr. Hooper started using mammography as a diagnostic tool in 1963 at Whitestone Hospital. To their surprise they were able to detect breast cancers that couldn't be felt. Other doctors started using mammography as the word got around the hospital about its usefulness. Opposition also developed.

Matt received a phone call from Bob Walker, the senior surgical cancer doctor at Whitestone Hospital.

"Matt, I wonder if you could come over to my office and discuss a matter of importance."

Matt replied, "I'll be right over."

As he walked over to the office he wondered what the matter of importance was. When he got to the office, the secretary told him to go right in to Dr. Walker's consultation room. Bob Walker was standing, waiting for him.

"Matt, I understand you and Paul Hooper are doing mammograms on quite a few breast patients."

"That's right. We've been doing them for over two years."

"Who gave you permission to do them?"

"No one. We looked up the literature and decided to try it out."

"Do you realize that you're exposing breasts to high doses of ionizing radiation?"

"It's about fifteen rads," said Matt. "If we pick up enough undetectable cancers, it will be worth it."

"You should have gone through the research committee," said Dr. Walker.

"It takes forever to get something through that research committee and anyway, you need a senior member of the staff to sponsor you."

"You shouldn't have gone off half cocked," said Walker.

"Well, how about you being our sponsor?"

"I don't approve of it. I won't sponsor you. You may get a bunch of lawsuits from those women on whom you don't detect breast cancer."

"Thanks a lot," said Matt as he walked out of the office.

He walked over to the chief surgeon's office, Dr. Jack Diamond, and told him about his plight.

"How many cases have you got?" asked Jack.

"About eighty."

"Get some of the best cases together and let me look at the x-rays with you."

Matt showed him some of his best cases and Jack was impressed.

"Have you documented all these cases?"

"Yes," he replied.

"I'll talk to Bob Walker. I don't think we want all the surgeons doing this until you're sure it's really helpful. It's too bad that so much radiation has to be used to get good pictures."

"I understand that they're developing new machines with less radiation exposure and that Kodak is developing better film for visualizing the tumors."

"Well, that would answer all our questions," replied Jack.

A year later, new mammography machines with less x-ray exposure were on the market.

Matt and Dr. Hooper wanted to have the x-ray department purchase one.

Three months later, Matt was eating breakfast with the chief resident, Dr. Phil Marks, and the surgical residents on his service before going into the operating room. He noticed a table in the center of the hospital cafeteria occupied by six to eight doctors. They were having their breakfast and conversing with Mr. Snow, the chief administrator of the hospital. The conversation seemed quite animated.

"Dr. Mark, what's that elite group of doctors doing over there?"

"Haven't you seen them before?"

"No," replied Matt.

"That's what the residents call the Inner Sanctum Brain Trust. Those guys are the head honchos of the medical establishment in this hospital."

"Hmm. That's interesting," said Matt. "The only one I recognize is Dr. Steve Walters, the young medical oncologist from Dana Farber Cancer Institute in Boston. I've had a couple of cases with him."

Just then, Dr. Walters got up and walked over to the table where Matt was sitting.

"Matt, Mr. Snow, our chief administrator, would like you to join our table for breakfast. He wants to pick your brain about something."

"I'd be glad to," he replied.

Matt was introduced to the various doctors seated around the table; Dr. Burns, the chief of urology; Dr. Milstein, the chief of neurosurgery; Dr. Andrews, a general practitioner and Dr. Alford, the chief of psychiatry.

"Matt, Dr. Walters tells me that you've been in the forefront of using x-ray to help detect cancers in the breast. I understand that you've been working with one of our radiology attendings in perfecting the technique," said Mr. Snow.

"That's right. Dr. Hooper and I have done quite a few patients and it really works."

"Any problems?"

"Yes. The breast is exposed to radiation."

"That's what I hear. Well, there's something new. Tom Bradley in purchasing told me that he was approached by one of the big corporations that has developed a new machine that does the same imaging with much less radiation exposure."

"That's great!" said Matt. "When are we going to get it?"

"That's the rub. We have to go to the hospital cost commission in order to get one. They're afraid the machine will be overutilized and just add to the cost of healthcare."

"That's bullshit! If we reduce the amount of radiation exposure to the breast we'll take the fear of doing the test away and we'll save more lives."

"Well, how would you like to go before the hospital cost commission and convince them of our need?"

"I'll be glad to do it," replied Matt.

Three weeks later, Matt went before the hospital cost commission and showed them three breast cancer cases that couldn't be felt but were detected by mammography.

A week later, the hospital was informed that they could buy the new machine.

12

WHEN MATT FIRST GOT BACK from New York City, most of the radical cancer surgery was being sent out of town, to Boston or New York. There was one surgeon, Dr. Walker, who did the remaining radical surgery.

It wasn't long before Dr. Kendall was referred complicated pelvic cases with multi-organ involvement. After doing a successful pelvic exenteration—resection of the uterus, colon and bladder with reconstruction—he was called into the chief gynecologist's office at Whitestone Hospital. He was told in no uncertain terms that he was not to do that type of surgery again.

"You should have called in a gynecologist when you saw the uterus was involved with cancer."

"Dr. Brooks, I was trained to do this type of case."

"I don't care how much training you've had or how good a surgeon you are. Those cases are to be controlled and done by gynecologists."

"Wait a minute," said Matt. "Am I hearing you correctly?"

Dr. Brooks pontificated that he had to protect his own boys and, although they had no one with the expertise to do the pelvic exenteration, they didn't want some young whippersnapper to get a reputation so he could become king of the hill. He said he'd rather send the cases to Boston or New York.

Matt felt great after having that conversation. In other words, you needed to have his blessing, the blessing of the gynecology chief, if you wanted to do the big multi-organ cases, even if the other surgeons in his department couldn't do them.

He decided to talk to the older cancer surgeon, Dr. Walker, who was referred some of the big cases. He was surprised by his reply. "I don't want to cut up the pie. You'll have to develop your own reputation," he said.

Walker told Matt that one of the reasons he was so upset was because Matt had his picture in the newspaper announcing the opening of his practice. The paper told about his war record as a navy night torpedo bomber pilot and his participation in the night carrier raids over Tokyo and Iwo Jima. It so happened that Dr. Walker had not gone to war during World War II. He was against the war philosophically and was deferred. He told Matt that he shouldn't have had his war record included in his bibliography in the newspaper.

"War has nothing to do with surgery. I agree. But character has a direct bearing on what kind of a surgeon a man is. You didn't serve. I did. I'm proud of risking my life for my country. If my patients are to trust me with their lives, they deserve to know who I am and what my background is."

"You're in the real world now," said Dr. Walker, "It's competitive and I don't want any competition. You're on your own. You're in a different war now."

"Thanks a lot."

A breakthrough for Matt finally came from the urology department. One of the senior urologists got into trouble trying to resect a large bladder cancer on a prominent local citizen. Dr. Walker was out of town. Dr. Kendall was doing a procedure in an adjacent operating room.

Mrs. Johnson, the OR supervisor, came into Matt's operating room as he was finishing his case.

"Dr. Kendall, Dr. Charles Marvel would like you to consult on a case that he's doing in room 507. He's having some problems."

"I'll be there as soon as I finish."

"Could you speed it up? He got into bleeding. He really needs your help right away."

"I'll be right there."

When he got to room 507, he quickly scrubbed up and put on a gown and gloves.

Dr. Marvel was obviously chasing a bleeder that he encountered while trying to resect a bladder cancer. The anesthesiologist was frantically pumping blood into the patient to replace the blood loss.

"I need help," said Charley, profusely sweating above his mask as he worked trying to find the bleeding point. Two metal suckers were screeching, draining the internal bleeding.

Matt had seen problems like this many times in New York City and he felt he knew what to do.

"Would you like me to take over?"

"Of course! This guy's bleeding to death," said Dr. Marvel.

"Let me have three or four heavy gauze lap pads," Matt said to the scrub nurse.

He took the bundle of pads and placed them in the pelvis where most of the bleeding was coming from and applied pressure. Using the metal suckers, he sucked the blood out around the pads. The bleeding was temporarily controlled.

"Tell me about the case," said Matt, as he compressed the bleeders.

"This man is a sixty-one-year-old insurance executive who noticed blood in his urine three weeks ago. I took a look inside his bladder and found a big cancer that I biopsied. Unfortunately, a few minutes ago I accidently cut a vein in the pelvis as I was trying to get around the tumor."

Matt continued to apply pressure.

"Get some arterial silk," he told the scrub nurse. "Do you have any vascular clamps, DeBakey clamps, or bulldog clamps on the table?"

"No," replied the scrub nurse.

"Get them! Right away!" He continued to apply pressure.

When the clamps arrived, Matt decided to remove the packs controlling the bleeding. He could see that there was a big hole in one of the large veins in the pelvis. He applied a vascular clamp and oversewed the hole and the bleeding stopped. Marvel looked on, embarrassed and ashen.

"I'll help you finish up the case if you want me to," offered Matt.

"Go right ahead," he replied.

Matt quickly dissected the tissues posteriorly to get the bladder tumor away from the colon, and slowly cut around the base. He cut the two ureters that brought the urine from the kidneys to the bladder and selected a segment of the distal small bowel in which to place the ends of the ureters. That segment of bowel would act as a reservoir to collect urine, and the patient would wear a bag on the abdominal wall. The procedure went well and the patient was sent home on the eleventh hospital day.

Word soon got around that Dr. Kendall knew how to do bladder resections. Dr. Whitney had trained him well in New York. Some senior urologists requested that he scrub on their cases. Eventually he was referred cases directly.

Some of the young urology residents asked if they could scrub on his bladder cancer cases and he encouraged them. As more and more of the young urologists became better trained in the more difficult procedures, the referral patterns changed.

13

"MATT," SAID JACK DIAMOND, the Chief of Surgery, "remember that liver case you helped me with when you were the chief surgical resident? We tried to resect the right lobe of the liver and the patient died on the table from blood loss."

"How can I forget that case? We blew it. We probably shouldn't have done that one."

"What do you mean?"

"That patient had severe cirrhosis of the liver. It was as hard as a rock, for God's sake. There was no way those blood vessels could have been occluded to stop bleeding."

"As it happens, I agree with you," said Diamond. "Did you work on any liver cases down in New York?"

"Yes, I did," said Matt. "That hospital's the center of radical surgery. There aren't any anatomical barriers to tackling a problem. I saw excellent, good, and poor liver surgery. The whole gamut."

"Did you learn any new tricks?"

"I learned to be very selective about which patients to operate on. The morbidity and mortality rate is very high, as high as 50 percent. In some hands, it's 100 percent."

"Most of the patients with cancer involving the liver are going to die within six months anyway," said Jack. "But you're right. The level of expertise ranges widely. What would you do if you developed a cancer of the liver involving one lobe? Would you go for it or would you try the chemotherapy route?"

"I wouldn't try chemotherapy. I worked with the experimental surgical group down there in New York. We did hepatic artery perfusions. We directed a catheter through the blood vessels to the liver and then gave a high dose of toxic drugs. Those patients just got sick and lost their hair. Some turned bright yellow from jaundice and they lived maybe three months longer. It costs a fortune. It wasn't cost effective!"

"What you're saying is there's no silver bullet."

"That's right."

"If you've got a solitary tumor in the liver, and the lungs and belly are free, I'd go for it. I'd have them cut it out."

"What sort of a work-up would you do?"

"I'd do a liver biopsy, if the patient wasn't a cirrhotic. I would want to see if the patient had a primary liver tumor or one that spread from the colon. I might also do a barium enema to make sure the colon was free."

"Who's doing most of the liver resections at Sloan now?" asked Jack.

"There are quite a few trying. The best are being done by George Packard. He's a virtuoso. He's terrifically gifted."

"Does he lose any patients from blood loss?"

"I haven't seen one."

"Who else?"

"Alexander Hart, but his technique is a bit rougher. He uses the guillotine approach. He puts this big cleaver, called the nitrogen knife, down through the liver and then uses a freezing coolant that he pours into the blade. It's like a witch's brew. When he removes the nitrogen knife, he then uses a lot of packs for compression against the raw liver surface. Five days later he takes the packs out. Sometimes the patients bleed and he loses them. One time I saw the nitrogen knife get frozen against the liver's raw surface. He had a difficult time getting that cleaver out of the patient's belly.' "

"Well, I guess I'll send the case down to George Packard," said Dr. Diamond.

"Why don't you let me see that patient?"

"I'll talk to him," said Jack. "Don't get your hopes up. He's a bigshot."

"They don't win them all down there in New York City. Or in Boston."

"Well, from our conversation, I know he needs a more complete work-up to see if he's eligible for a resection."

"If he decides to have it done here, you can assist me doing the resection. It takes two people to do a good one."

"What do you mean?"

"Well, the liver has a tight capsule around it—a fibrous covering. George Packard usually does a finger fractionating technique, or uses the metal-tip sucker to pick up the larger blood vessels in the liver because it's so soft.

"He then suture ligates the big blood vessels as he cuts through the liver. Sometimes he uses blunt-tipped liver needles that he passes through the liver, and then ties the heavy suture down to compress the tissue and control the bleeding."

"Have you worked on livers in the dog lab?" asked Jack.

"Yes. I've been working with one of our chief residents. We've practiced on four or five dogs over there."

"Do the dogs die?"

"No," said Matt. "They're under anesthesia during the surgery, and their livers regenerate."

"Well, I'm going to give it some thought as to whether we send the case down to New York or whether we do it up here. I'll be in touch," said Jack.

About a week later, Matt received a call from Dr. Diamond.

"That patient I talked to you about is in the hospital. He wants to meet you. His name is Bill Hartman and he's on North Ten."

After he finished office hours, Matt went up to North Ten, on the Gold Coast. He walked into Bill Hartman's room. There he saw a tall, thin, white male about 65 years of age with gray hair and brilliant green eyes. He was sitting in a chair, reading a novel.

"I'm Dr. Matt Kendall," he said as he held out his hand.

"Yes, I know," said the gentleman. "I could tell by the way you came in and the way you walked. Dr. Diamond tells me you're an ex navy pilot. You look like a man who has a lot of confidence. I can tell you're an aggressive guy, too."

"How can you tell that?"

"You charged right in here and you didn't bother to knock on the door."

OK, thought Matt. This guy's pretty sharp.

"Dr. Diamond tells me you had a colon resection three years ago and now you have trouble in your liver. Have you lost any weight?"

"Not really," replied Mr. Hartman. "I've always been thin. I jog every day and watch what I eat."

"How much did Dr. Diamond tell you about the problem you have with your liver?"

"He was very frank. I believe he told me everything. Evidently, a piece of that tumor in my colon broke off and it's lodged in the right lobe of my liver. They did a needle biopsy two days ago and he told me the biopsy of the tissue shows it's related to my colon. As far as he could tell, there's no other area in my body that's involved right now."

"Did he discuss what should be done about it?"

"Yes. He told me I could do nothing and I'd probably live for six months. I also have the choice of taking systemic chemotherapy drugs to try to suppress the growth of the tumor. It would make me quite sick. Or I could have surgery. He said you were one of the young surgeons who had the most experience in doing this type of surgery. He said you were from Sloan Kettering. He also gave me the option of going there for the surgery."

"What did you decide?"

"I'm a New England Yankee, so I've decided to take my chances in New England. I don't like the Big Apple."

"Good," said Matt. "We'll do our best."

When he got back to his office, he called the animal lab and scheduled two dogs to be done. He also called the chief resident surgeon, who was elated; he also wanted to learn how to do the operation.

Matt called a gastroenterologist to see Mr. Hartman in consultation to see if his patient's medical perimeters were okay for surgery. He ordered a battery of chemistry tests and checked to see if his blood clotted well.

Matt talked to Dr. Diamond the day before the surgery. "Do you want to assist?"

"No, Matt, you and the chief resident can do the case. I'll be available if you need any help."

The day finally arrived. Matt had talked to the OR supervisor to make sure that all the special vascular clamps, such as the DeBakeys, would be available. He also requested an experienced scrub nurse to assist.

The chief resident surgeon lined up a big intern to hold the retractors for exposing the area to be operated on. The large amphitheater was secured for the surgery and the chief of anesthesia and two of his residents would be in charge of putting the patient out and monitoring any fluid or blood loss.

When the patient was being wheeled into the operating room, Dr. Shea, the chief of anesthesia, spoke to Matt. "We'll have to put a central venous line in. What's your anticipated blood loss?"

"Probably six to eight units."

"We'll check with the blood bank to be sure they're available."

Finally, the patient was prepped and draped after the endotracheal tube was placed in the throat.

The scalpel was given to Dr. Kendall and he made a large incision through the skin and musculature of the upper abdomen. He explored the abdomen by hand to be sure there were no other abdominal tumors. After a short while, he found a seven-inch white cancerous tumor penetrating right through the mid-surface of the right lobe of the liver.

When he determined there were no other cancers, he carried the incision through the ribs and the diaphragm muscle was cut up to the undersurface of the heart. Cloth packs were placed behind the liver so that the liver surface could be worked on easier. Because the patient was thin, the exposure was excellent.

Matt quickly removed the gallbladder and the duct that drains the bile from the liver was exposed. He sharply dissected around it up into the liver. The bile duct that drained the right lobe was doubly tied with silk. The right hepatic artery and right hepatic vein were isolated and tied. This was done to prevent blood from going into or coming out of the right lobe of the liver.

On the undersurface of the liver, the large vein (inferior vena cava) that returns most of the blood from the lower part of the body to the heart was isolated. Vascular tapes were placed around it, one above and one below the liver. The vein was about the size of a large sausage.

Matt then sharply incised the thick covering around the liver, named the Glisson's capsule, in the midline. He then used finger dissection, the back of the scalpel and, at one point, the sharp tip of the blood sucker to cut through the liver tissue. Some of the smaller blood vessels were cut and vascular clips were used to control the bleeding. The large vessels were sutured with silk. The liver was then retracted upward to expose the small hepatic veins that drain into the vena cava, which goes to the heart. During the procedure, Matt and his team continued to work fast to minimize the blood loss. The right lobe of the liver was removed, drains were placed in the upper abdomen, and the specimen was checked to make sure adequate margins were obtained.

Matt and his chief resident surgeon had been working for five hours. He finally looked up as the specimen was removed. Dr. Diamond was standing behind him, looking over his shoulder.

"That was a good job," he said. "I think that patient is going to make it."

Diamond had been quietly standing there for a long time.

Matt looked over at the chief anesthesiologist. "How much blood did we lose?"

"Six units, Matt. The patient's blood pressure never went below 100."

Two weeks later Mr. Hartman was discharged from the hospital. Before he left he spoke to Matt. "I knew you could do it. But you didn't tell me that Whitestone Hospital hadn't had much success in the past with liver resections."

"If I had told you, would it have made a difference?"

"Sure. I would have worried a little bit more. I might have gone to New York. Now I can tell everyone that I was one of the first successful liver resections done at Whitestone Hospital."

14

IN THE SURGEON'S LOUNGE, Matt was relaxing with the morning newspaper between his surgical cases.

Jack Diamond walked in and said, "I want to talk to you about that argument you had a few weeks ago at the morbidity and mortality conference with Dr. Dakin, our renowned thoracic surgeon."

"I prefer to think of it as a mildly heated discussion."

"I'll bet you do."

Dr. Dakin had presented a case of a 50-year-old male, who had a cancer of the distal esophagus, the tube that goes from the mouth to the stomach. He developed a leak from the anastomosis—where the two ends were put together—between the distal esophagus and the stomach. The patient was very sick and nearly died. Dr. Dakin, one of the senior thoracic surgeons, had trained in Boston and bragged that he was getting 40 percent five-year survival rates with his surgical esophageal cases. Matt had challenged him in the conference and Dr. Dakin had made some snide remarks about the fact that the New York surgeons never did learn how to do that operation properly.

Matt blasted him, saying that if you select the cases with the smallest tumors, you could possibly get a 15 percent five-year survival rate. But 40 percent? Fantasy.

Dakin blew his stack. "If you don't know what you're talking about, you shouldn't speak up at these conferences."

"Present some documentation," Matt had shouted, "if the data backs you up."

Dakin's face and neck turned crimson. Who did this insolent young upstart think he was? "When you've been around here a little bit longer, we'll listen to your heroics."

Dr. Diamond, who was moderating the meeting, stepped in

abruptly and said, "Enough. We don't need arguments in here. We don't want you two guys coming to blows." He then turned to the chief resident surgeon and said, "Let's go on to the next complication."

Matt Kendall looked up from his newspaper, looked Dr. Diamond straight in the eyes, smiled a weak smile, and replied. "I didn't agree with my learned colleague's comments about the treatment of esophageal cancer."

"I know," said Jack. "I didn't agree either."

"You can't do a good en bloc resection of the tumor and get around the tumor totally with the heart and lungs right there. In fact, I talked to the people over at the State Tumor Registry and asked them to pull all the esophageal cancer cases that were cured in the last ten years. There were only sixty cases alive out of one-thousand. That's only six percent."

"That follows with my experience, too," said Dr. Diamond.

"The issue is how to palliate these people successfully. They drown in their own mucous secretions and can't swallow food, let alone enjoy it."

"That's what I want to talk to you about," said Jack. "What are they doing down in New York that we're not doing here?"

"A few things," said Matt. "They're resecting the esophagus and then using the right colon to replace it. They make a tunnel under the sternum and hook the colon up in the neck. Below, they hook it up to the stomach. The patients can swallow food and the mucus doesn't go into the lungs."

"Do you think you could do one?" asked Jack.

"Sure. But you've got to get the case first."

"Consider it done."

"Who and where?"

"Mr. Willard. He's on Center 10. I told him about you."

"I'll see him after I finish my morning schedule."

That afternoon, Matt went up to see Mr. Willard. The man was relaxing in a lounge chair in his bathrobe, reading a book. He told Matt that he had been a successful businessman, owned a small tool shop, made airplane parts, and had 31 employees in his company. He was also a heavy smoker and drinker and was now retired.

"I drank a lot of white lightning in my days," he said. "I bought a lot of white lightning for the purchasing agents at the aircraft factory in order to get more business for my tool shop. I can't drink anymore. It burns like hell going down. I've also lost forty pounds in the past six months. I can't swallow anything. And I can't spit up. I'm miserable and I don't want to die like this."

"Well, you do have a serious problem. You have a cancer obstructing the tube that goes from your mouth to your stomach. That's why you've lost so much weight."

Matt stopped talking for a minute and then said, "Mr. Willard, there are a lot of different ways to approach your problem. You can have extensive surgery, radiation treatment, chemotherapy, all three, or nothing."

"Let's be realistic about this," said Mr. Willard. "I know I'm going to die. But before I die, I'd like to swallow some food and maybe a few martinis. Is there any operation you can do so I'll be able to swallow comfortably?"

"I believe there is. We can make a new tube that will go from your mouth to your stomach by using part of your colon. It's extensive surgery and it's risky."

"Some of my friends have had chemotherapy. They vomit and lose their hair," said Mr. Willard. "I don't plan to go that route. I'd take a morphine drip before taking all that poison. I don't think they ever cure anybody with those chemicals. I'm willing to take my chances on surgery. Do you have to do any more tests?"

"Just one more. We'll have to do a barium enema to make sure your colon is open and free of disease."

"Well, let's get on with it. Do I have to sign anything?"

"Yes," said Matt as he handed him a clipboard with a pink sheet.

Mr. Willard signed the informed-consent form without reading it.

"Do you have any questions?"

"No, just one request," said Mr. Willard. "Make sure you get a good night's sleep before you do my operation. I don't want any foul-ups."

Three days later, Matt and Jack Diamond operated on Mr. Willard. Two senior surgical residents assisted.

Jack started working in the belly, freeing up the colon, while Matt entered the chest to resect the esophagus. A tunnel was made under the sternum, to put in the colon which was hooked up to the esophagus in the neck. Blood loss was minimal. Because the patient had lost so much weight, it was easy to do the operation. It took approximately six hours.

About ten days after the operation, the patient was given some barium to swallow to see if the connections between the esophagus and the stomach were intact. They were.

The chest tubes and drains were removed and the patient was given food to eat for the first time in six months: Jello, cereal, and eggs.

Three days later, he had a normal bowel movement. The man was ecstatic, and he was discharged from the hospital.

"I think I'll be able to swallow my white lightning without up-chucking. I'm going to celebrate."

"I wouldn't overdo it."

After Mr. Willard went home, Matt and the resident staff were euphoric. The first colon substitution for esophageal cancer at White-stone had been successful. The patient had been discharged in two weeks. Word quickly got around that there was another way of treating esophageal cancer. Dr. Dakin, the chest surgeon, was furious.

A 2 A.M., the night after Mr. Willard was discharged, Matt and his wife were sound asleep when the phone rang. Nancy answered the phone.

"Dr. Kendall's residence," she said groggily.

A woman's voice blurted out, "My husband, my husband—he's dead."

"Who is this?"

"Mrs. Willard, Mrs. Willard."

"Hold on for a minute."

She shook Matt and woke him up. "There's a woman on the phone, screaming. She's frantic. She said her husband's dead."

"What's her name?" asked Matt as he rubbed his eyes.

"A Mrs. Willard."

Matt sat bolt upright in bed. "Oh no, oh no, I can't believe it!" he gasped. "What happened?"

"I don't know," replied Nancy. "She didn't tell me. She's on the phone."

"Damn it," said Matt as the color started to drain from his face. "This is horrible. He was doing so well." He reached over and took the phone from his wife.

"Mrs. Willard, this is Dr. Kendall. Tell me what happened."

"My husband just got home from the hospital. I haven't seen him all day. He came into the living room and dropped dead right in front of me."

Matt was trying to control his emotions. "What can I do?" he asked.

"I don't know what to do." she said frantically.

"Call Dr. Eliot, your family doctor. Tell him everything. I'm not familiar with the area where you live. I'm sorry this happened."

"So am I," said Mrs. Willard. "He was doing so well in the hospital." She wept as she spoke, gasping for air through her sobs.

"If you can't get Dr. Eliot, call me right back."

"I will."

Matt waited, but the phone never rang. He lay in bed, crushed. For God's sake, that man was *alive* when he left the hospital and he was *smiling*. Matt went through the operation over and over in his mind, remembering every cut, each stitch. Then he worried that there could be a malpractice suit. It was a new experimental operation. Although he had talked at length with Mr. and Mrs. Willard about the procedure and its risks, Mr. Willard had said he would take them. The man knew his fate. What he really wanted was to improve the quality of his life— the ability to swallow.

"Try to get some sleep," said Nancy. "You've got another big day ahead of you. You know in your heart you tried your best."

He finally fell asleep around 4:00 A.M. At 5:00 A.M. the phone rang again.

"It's probably Mrs. Willard again," he said. "She probably couldn't get Dr. Eliot."

He picked up the phone.

"This is Dr. Kendall."

"Matt, this is Dr. Eliot. Don't you ever call me in the middle of the night to pronounce a patient of yours dead!"

"I'm sorry, Dr. Eliot, but I don't know that Park Street area of town, particularly at night."

He heard a repressed laugh at the other end of the phone. What the hell was going on? Then, in a stern voice, Dr. Eliot said, "Don't ever pull that stunt on me again!"

"I'm sorry," said Matt. "I would have gone myself, but I—"

"—Matt, I can't stand this rhetoric anymore. Relax. Mr. Willard is not dead! He drank a barrel full of martinis. He got drunk as a hoot owl and passed out in the middle of his living room. His blood pressure, pulse and everything are normal. He's sleeping soundly in his bed."

Stunned, Matt stammered, "What the . . . you son of a . . . that's great! I owe you one."

A week later, when Mr. Willard came into Matt's office for follow-up, he had a sheepish grin on his face.

"You almost gave me a goddamned heart attack. What happened?"

"Well," he said, "when I got out of the hospital, I took a cab to that fancy restaurant in the South End. You know the one—The Hearth-stone. The one that serves those great big steaks. I ordered the biggest one in the house since I hadn't really eaten in six months. I also had ten dry Martinis, straight up. The rest is history."

"Great," said Matt. "I thought *you* were history."

"Dr. Kendall, I want to thank you," said Willard. "Lighten up. You fulfilled your part of the bargain. That was the best steak I ever ate."

15

UNKNOWN TO THE PUBLIC, there is intense competition in this country for the limited number of head and neck cancer patients. This competition has intensified in recent years. Surgical oncologists trained in head and neck surgery, in New York City and Texas and other centers, now compete with plastic surgeons, ear, nose and throat surgeons, and more recently, oral surgeons who also have their M.D.

Some of these experts can do a good neck dissection but usually cannot handle the complications that occasionally develop in difficult cases, particularly vascular problems, where bleeding, persistent fistulas, or severe cosmetic defects can make a straightforward case complex. In some centers this has led to the multidisciplinary surgical approach to head and neck cancer, in which the case is shared between two or more surgeons.

When Dr. Kendall returned to Whitestone from New York City, he knew he would be competing with these specialists. He felt that working with the doctors on the head and neck service at Sloan Kettering had prepared him for doing good head and neck cancer surgery.

Soon Matt began to operate on the more difficult cases, doing laryngectomies with neck dissections, tongue, mandible, and neck dissections, and resections of tumors of the salivary glands and maxillary sinuses.

The operating room personnel noticed that many of the difficult procedures were being done with minimal loss of blood, and so he earned the nickname "Mr. Clean."

One morning the phone rang in Dr. Kendall's bedroom at 5 A.M. His wife picked up the phone.

"Dr. Kendall's residence."

"This is Dr. Malcolm Dole. I'd like to talk to Dr. Kendall. Is he home?"

"Yes," she said. She recognized his name. Dr. Dole was the Chief of the Oral Surgery Department at the hospital. He had an M.D. from Harvard and a dental degree and was well respected by the hospital staff. "Dr. Dole wants to talk to you, Matt." He rubbed his eyes and took the phone.

"Hi, Mal. What's on your mind?"

"Matt, we have a problem that we need your help with."

"What's the problem?"

"We have a three-year-old girl who's bleeding massively from her upper palate area. We don't know what's going on."

"What happened?"

"Her mother took her to a pediatrician who referred her to our office. She had been bleeding intermittently from the left upper molar area and was taken to a dentist's office and one of her upper molars was hanging free in the breeze, so to speak. There was quite a bit of bleeding, so when the dentist saw this he brought her over to our oral surgery office. We brought her here immediately. When we got her into the emergency room she stopped bleeding. We took x-rays that showed some bone erosion of the left upper palate. The left maxillary sinus is filled with opaque material. Our plan was to work her up but she started to bleed about an hour ago. One of the oral surgical residents is holding pressure on the bleeding area right now."

"How old did you say she was?"

"Three years old," replied Dr. Dole.

"Call the chief resident on the surgical service and have him put a cutdown in so we can replace the blood loss. I'll be in as fast as I can."

Matt dressed and sped to the hospital. When he arrived, the patient was already in the operating room. He quickly changed into his operating room attire and put on his gown and gloves. There was no time for a scrub. The child was in shock and they were pumping blood into one of her veins through a cutdown in the ankle area. He took over as soon as he entered the room.

The oral surgical resident was as white as a sheet holding his forefinger in the hole of the tooth socket.

"I need a quick look. Take your hand out."

When he did, a fountain of bright red arterial blood shot out of the mouth. Matt quickly put his finger in the hole and had the resident suck out the blood. The child was terrified and struggled weakly.

There was a good young anesthesiologist at the head of the operating table who Matt knew could handle difficult pediatric airway problems.

"Do you think you can get an endotracheal tube down her throat with my finger in the dike?" he asked Nick.

"I can give it a try," he replied.

"Good. Put her under."

Nick took his pediatric laryngoscope and put it in the child's mouth. There was a lot of blood-tinged mucous in the back of her throat.

"We've got to suck this stuff out of her throat so I can see where I'm going," said Nick. "Come on, dammit, give me some help!" The suction apparatus was put into the mouth.

Then, using a long, thin pediatric anesthesia tube, he lifted up on the chin with his left hand, exposing, what he thought were the vocal chords, and slid the tube in with his right hand.

"Listen to the chest to see if I'm in," he said as he squeezed the bag.

"Sounds good," said one of the other anesthesiologists.

Matt sucked out the clot and debris in the left upper palate area and put a large Iodoform packing in the defect to control the bleeding.

He then made a small incision over the major artery in the left upper neck. Using sharp and blunt dissection, he isolated the external carotid artery, the main blood vessel that went to the area of the palate and jaw. He tied the large artery off with silk.

The bleeding slowed down dramatically. He could now see more clearly what was going on in the mouth. He removed the packing. The bone was eroded in the palate area and two other molars were hanging loosely. He removed these to get access to the bleeding in the left maxillary sinus. He then cut directly into the sinus using the cautery and special instruments. He used multiple suture ligatures to tie off the blood vessels. He removed the clots from the sinus and cauterized the bleeding points and quickly excised a large polypoid tumor. He took another iodoform pack and packed the sinus and molar area, tightly placing sutures around the tissue and tying them over the packing to apply pressure. The bleeding stopped.

A tracheostomy was done in the midline lower neck because the packing filled a good part of the mouth and the child wouldn't be able to breathe without the airway opening in the neck.

Five days later, the child was taken back to the operating room, the packing was removed, and the left upper neck skin sutures were taken out. The breathing tube was taken out three days later. The analysis of the bone and tissues came back as a benign blood vessel polypoid fibrous tumor.

The patient had no further problems.

Dr. John Wise, an anesthesiologist, came into the operating room.

"Dr. Kendall, may I interrupt?"

"What's up?"

"Dr. Phil Weiner is doing a head and neck case next door in Room 155—a parotid salivary gland tumor. He's having difficulty locating the facial nerve. He'd like you to spare a minute or two to help him out."

"How long has he been working?"

"About four hours."

"Well, I'm pretty much through here. The residents can put a chest tube in and sew up the chest wall. Tell him I'll be in there in about five minutes."

Matt took his gown and gloves off, left the operating room, and walked down the hall to room 155. He put on a new cap and mask and walked into the room.

Dr. Weiner had made the proper type of incision to explore the parotid gland in front of the left ear, but he obviously had gotten nowhere in finding the facial nerve that goes through the gland.

Standing on a high stool behind Dr. Weiner was John Russell, one of the senior anesthesiologists. He was trying to tell him where to look for the nerve. He kept saying, "It starts closer to the ear."

"Phil, what's the problem?"

"I've got a tough one here," he said. "This patient's got a lump in his parotid gland and I can't find the facial nerve."

"What sort of a work-up has he had?" asked Matt.

"I did an ultrasound of the gland."

Matt could see the small, egg-sized mass next to the ear.

"Did he have anything in his mouth?"

"Nothing that I could see," replied Phil.

"Anything unusual about his history?"

"Not too much. He does smoke and drinks whiskey occasionally."

"Hmm. Do you want me to scrub up and help you?"

"I'd appreciate it."

Matt went into the scrub room and did a five-minute scrub. He put on a new gown and gloves and returned to the OR. First he felt the exposed neck.

"Did you feel anything in the upper neck?"

"There was some fullness," said Weiner.

"I thought there were some glands," said Dr. Jones, an assistant surgical resident.

"I think there are, too," replied Matt.

"Do you want me to help you find the facial nerve?"

"Yes."

"First I have to tell you, you haven't gotten through the capsule of the gland. That's one reason why you can't find the nerve. You have to dissect deeper. The nerve sort of bisects the gland. I use an old trick that Dr. Hayes showed me in New York. He would dissect down the outside of the ear canal and then he'd put his forefinger against the canal and, sure enough, the nerve would be right there every time."

Matt quickly dissected with the Metzenbaum surgical scissors and lo and behold, there was the nerve. It took him about 20 minutes. He quickly worked around the tumor and removed it.

He then dissected in the upper neck. "Listen, Phil, I think this patient may have a cancer. We'll give the pathologist one of these lymph glands to look at, too."

He quickly removed a lymph node. "Call the pathologist. I think we'd better see what the parotid tumor and that lymph gland shows before we do anything more."

About ten minutes later, the pathologist came into the operating room.

"That parotid gland and lymph node have squamous cell cancer in them."

"Well, Phil, what do you want to do now?"

"I don't know," he replied. "I'm open to your suggestions."

"He needs his throat looked at more closely. Do you have permission to do a radical neck dissection?"

"No," replied Dr. Weiner.

"Well, then I'd close him up and complete the work-up. You'll have to tell him what happened. He may need another operation."

"Thanks for your help. I appreciate it."

Matt sensed that he did.

★ ★ ★

Matt usually had breakfast with Nancy before going to the hospital. Sometimes the conversation was about medical problems of friends that Nancy wanted to discuss with him.

"Matt, I want to talk to you about Sally Lord's husband, Bob. She's a friend of mine from church."

"What's wrong with him?"

"He's in Carlisle Hospital and he's deathly sick. Sally's a basket case. Evidently Bob was operated on for nasal polyps three days ago and they told her he's an alcoholic. He's having DTs in their intensive care unit. He's had to be tied down and restrained."

"I didn't know Bob was an alcoholic. The last time we played bridge with them he hardly had anything to drink."

"He's not, according to his wife. They each have a glass of wine at night before dinner, but no whiskey."

"That's not being an alcoholic! You're not telling me everything. There's got to be more to the story."

"Well, you know that Bob's a vice president of an insurance company. His secretary was having some nasal obstruction and breathing difficulties so she went to a nose and throat specialist and he told her that she had nasal polyps. She went into Carlisle Hospital and had them removed. Her doctor told her that he just plucked them out like grapes. When she came back to the office she told Bob that she felt great. She could now breathe fresh air and had no more nasal obstruction. Bob decided to go see her doctor, since he also had problems breathing and thought he might also have nasal polyps.

"He went to see Dr. Dubinski, the ENT specialist, who looked into his nose and told him he did have nasal polyps. He then said, 'It'll be a piece of cake.'

"Well, it was a piece of cake, all right. Bob's in the Carlisle intensive care unit now and they say he's got DTs and might die."

"What do you want me to do about it, Nancy? Maybe he drinks when Sally's not around. He could be a closet drinker."

"I don't believe it. Would you talk to Sally?"

"If it will make you feel better, I'll be glad to."

"Great! I'll call her right now."

When Sally got on the phone she was crying. Matt decided to ask her some questions.

"Was there any problem during the operation? What did the doctor find?"

"I don't know," Sally replied. "The doctor did say that he bled quite a bit. Would you be able to see Bob?"

"I can't, unless you tell his doctor that you want me to see him. I don't have privileges at Carlisle. It's unethical for me to just barge in."

"Dr. Dubinski has told me nothing except that Bob's an alcoholic and that's why he's having all this trouble. I'll insist that I want you to see him."

"All right. Call me back after you talk to the doctor."

That afternoon, Matt got a call from Sally.

"I talked to Dr. Dubinski and he said he'd leave a note on Bob's chart so you could see him. He said he's got a temperature and that he's not doing too well. He's not sure what's going on. He's on the critical list."

"I'll drive down to Carlisle just as soon as I finish office hours," said Matt.

Carlisle Hospital was a small 300-bed hospital 20 miles from White-stone. As soon as Matt's patients were seen for the day, he drove there and went to the intensive care unit. He talked to the head nurse, Mrs. Simpson.

"I'm Dr. Matt Kendall, a friend of the Lords, and Mrs. Lord has asked me to see her husband. What's going on with him?"

"He's very sick. Dr. Dubinski thinks he's an alcoholic and has DTs. He actually started out as a minor case having polyps taken out of his nose. Then he became violent and had to be restrained. He's out of it. He's irrational and running a low-grade temp."

Matt went in and looked at Bob Lord. He was glassy-eyed and didn't recognize him and was straining at his restraints. Matt then looked at the chart at the nurses' station, which revealed nothing.

"Has the tissue diagnosis come back yet?" he asked Mrs. Simpson.

"No. It should be back within a day or two."

"Do you have Dr. Dubinski's number? I'd like to give him a call."

Matt was given the number and he called Dr. Dubinski. He got very little information from him, except that he felt there was excessive bleeding at the time of the operation.

The next morning, Matt mentioned the case to the doctors at White-stone while he was having coffee. Dr. Milstein, the neurosurgeon, spoke up.

"I'll bet that when he took those nasal polyps out, he got into the cribiform plate in the frontal lobe of the brain. Does he have any clear liquid coming from his nose?"

"Now that you mention it, I think he does."

"Well, he's probably leaking spinal fluid, then."

That evening Dr. Milstein drove to Carlisle Hospital, at Matt's request.

Bob was transferred to Whitestone Hospital by ambulance, where it was determined that Dr. Dubinski had gotten into the frontal lobe of his brain with his nasal instruments and perforated the cribiform plate in the back of the nose. That explained his confusion and leakage of spinal fluid.

A brain operation was done to patch the leak. It was successful. However, the frontal lobe of his brain had been damaged.

Bob Lord had an unplanned pre-frontal lobotomy which has been used in the past to calm down mentally disturbed patients. He got well—but not completely well. He lost his vigorous energy, libido, and became a zombie. He was relieved of his job as vice president at the insurance company. The case ended up in the courts and was settled for big bucks.

The payoff came when the analysis of the tissue from the original surgery showed that there were no polyps in the tissue removed from Bob's nose.

16

"HOW ARE THINGS GOING, anyway?" Jack asked. "You must be doing all right. I see you're booking three or four cases a day on the OR schedule."

"I'm paying the rent. I can't complain, although I'd really like to be doing more head and neck surgery. I really like that anatomical area of the body. It's a tough place to operate.

"Some general surgeons, ear, nose, and throat, and plastic surgeons don't know what they're doing when they work in the head and neck area. They haven't had enough specialized head and neck training in a cancer center."

"I know you're right," said Jack. "I just reviewed a case done by one of our fair-haired ENT surgeons that became a real tragedy."

"What happened?"

"Well, keep what I tell you under your hat. Our hospital is being sued for half a million dollars because of the ineptitude of this guy. I told the insurance company to pay the bill. It was Dr. John Cruse, one of our New York City-trained ENT doctors. He pulled a big boo-boo."

"What happened?"

"He scheduled a radical neck dissection on one of our local big-shots. Evidently, he hasn't done many radical neck operations. I think he does about one a year, if that. It turned out to be a bloody mess. The resident told me he didn't know where he was most of the time."

"What went wrong?"

"Well, when Dr. Cruse tried to isolate the internal jugular in the lower neck to tie it off, he tore a big hole in it. He tried to stitch it up, and after a loss of ten units of blood, he called for help from one of our senior vascular surgeons, Tom Young. Jim Kask, the man giving the anesthesia, was mad as hell and had to pump blood to maintain the blood pressure.

"Young scrubbed up to help out. He told me there were clamps all over the place in the wound—Kelly clamps, Halstead clamps, De-Bakey clamps, you name it. Cruse's voice was quite tremulous trying to describe to Young what happened.

"Young had done vascular surgery in the neck before on his vascular cases but he had never done any radical cancer surgery. That's a whole new ball of wax. He had trouble trying to figure out what was going on. The patient was critical after all that blood loss and there was still a lot of blood coming from the neck.

"Dr. Young told me what transpired when he got into the operating room.

" 'You got a mess here,' " said Young. " 'What started all this bleeding?' "

" 'I think I tore a hole in the internal jugular vein,' Cruse said. 'I clamped it immediately but it started bleeding profusely all over the place. I must have missed the bleeding point. The vein retracted under the collarbone so I held pressure on it so the patient wouldn't get an air embolis.' "

"Dr. Young called over the drapes to the anesthesiologist, 'You'd better type and cross-match three or four more units of blood.'

" 'He's had fourteen so far,' replied the anesthesiologist. 'You guys better get your act together and stop this bleeding.'

" 'Get another suction apparatus,' Young hollered to the circulating nurse. 'This one's plugged. I can't see what's going on here. Pump more blood into him to maintain his pressure.' "

Diamond paused, shaking his head. Then he continued to relate what happened. " 'We may have to split the clavicle to get better control of this blood vessel,' said Young. 'Do we have any bone-cutting instruments on board?'

" 'No,' said Cruse.

"Young called out to Sally, the circulating nurse, 'Go get some vascular clamps and bone cutters from my vascular room.' Finally, by using two suction devices, Young was able to suck out enough blood to see where it originated. He placed a vascular clamp across the hole and the bleeding slowed.

"He then began methodically to tie off the clamps in the neck, using arterial silk. The bleeding came under control as he tied and clamped each vessel. Luckily, he didn't have to cut through the collarbone.

"That's when the big mistake showed up.

"One of the large Kelly clamps, unfortunately, had been placed across part of the brachial plexus."

"Wait," interjected Matt. "Are you sure? My God! That nerve supplies motor function to the arm."

"Right," said Jack. "So Young said, 'We have a big problem here. This doesn't look too good. Better call one of the neurosurgeons in to see if we should do anything more about that brachial plexus nerve that you clamped. Sally, get Dr. White in here.' "

Diamond looked at Matt, whose contempt for this incompetence showed on his face. Jack continued, "So Young said to the neurosurgeon, 'Dr. Cruse inadvertently clamped part of the brachial plexus to control bleeding, and we've done nothing but release the clamp. Do you have any suggestions as to how to handle this problem?'

"Dr. White looked into the neck wound where the clamps had been placed. He paused for a while and then spoke: " 'Well, to be honest with you, I've never faced this problem before. The blood supply to that part of the nerve may be destroyed. How long was the clamp on for?'

'You'll have to ask Dr. Cruse that question,' said Young.

" 'Maybe twenty to forty minutes, I think. Possibly longer, replied Cruse.'

" 'I never heard of a nerve graft ever being put in that location. The blood supply to that part of the nerve may be destroyed. I think you have to leave the area alone and hope for the best. Wait and see what happens. Those blood vessels around the nerves are too small to try to repair.'

"The neck wound was then closed by Dr. Young and Dr. Cruse. Suction drains were put in the lower neck. When the patient woke up from the anesthesia, he couldn't move some of his fingers."

"Did he get return of function?" asked Matt.

"No," said Diamond. "At least not yet. It's been over a year."

"Was that worth half a million dollars?"

"I'd say so," said Jack. "He was left-handed. If it was you, you'd sue for five million dollars because you're a surgeon and you like to play golf, right?"

"Partially," said Matt. "I'd sue the reckless bastard because he had no business doing an operation he wasn't qualified to do."

★ ★ ★

"Bob Gold, the oral surgeon, is on the phone," said Judy.

"What does he want?" asked Matt.

"He's got a bigshot with what he thinks is a cancer of the lip. He wants you to see him right away."

"Work him into my schedule tomorrow afternoon. Who is he?"

"Donald Kelly."

"The former Democratic National Chairman? The guy that smokes cigars all the time?"

"None other," she replied.

"Set it up."

The next day, he examined Donald Kelly in the office. He had developed a raw area on the lower surface of his right lip where he often held his cigars. It looked like an obvious cancer of the lip to Matt. His throat also looked raw from the repeated irritations from the cigar smoke.

"Well, Mr. Chairman, I'm afraid you're going to need an operation on your lower lip."

"Will I need to go into the hospital?"

"Yes. I want to check the margins of the tissue resection while we're doing it," he replied.

"I'm a diabetic," said Mr. Kelly.

"Do you take insulin?"

"Yes," he replied.

"Well, don't take any insulin before you come into the hospital. You can't have anything to eat after midnight. The anesthesiologist will give you intravenous insulin and control your sugar that way, if necessary."

The next week, a biopsy of the lip lesion was done. It was a bad cancer, and Matt was able to get around it with adequate surgical margins. He was able to do it without disfiguring the man's lip.

Matt spoke to him after the operation. "You're going to have to quit smoking cigars."

Kelly was ready. "Can't do it, Doc. I've got a closet full of the best Havana cigars. They're worth a fortune and it's the most relaxing thing in my life."

"Your whole throat looks lousy. There's no telling where or when you'll get another cancer in your oral cavity. I'd quit if I were you. That cigar smoke is irritating the mucous membranes of your whole mouth cavity."

"I'll take that under advisement," said Kelly.

"That's the first time you've sounded like a politician," said Matt, and Kelly smiled. "Because your mouth looks so terrible, you should come in to see me every three months. The cancer of the lip I excised can travel into the glands in your neck, and you're at risk to develop a new cancer in your throat."

"That's the first time you've sounded like a doctor. Don't worry, I'll be here," he said, as he rolled his eyes and looked up at the ceiling.

That was the last time Matt saw him for quite a while.

He finally came back two years later, complaining of a sore throat. Using a bright light and mirror Matt was able to look in the back of his throat. He had developed a new tumor. He took a biopsy under local anesthesia and a few days later it came back positive. Matt had his secretary call Mr. Kelly and ask him to come into the office.

"You have a serious problem that has developed in your throat."

"What do you mean?"

"You've developed a new cancer."

"What do I do now?" asked Kelly.

"You've got three choices," he said to Mr. Kelly. "One, you can have radical surgery, which would include partial removal of your jawbone; two, you can have radiation therapy; or three, do nothing."

"I can't have radical surgery. I wouldn't look very good on television. I'll take the x-ray treatment."

"I'll set it up. They'll be giving you treatments over a course of approximately five weeks. You'll be treated every day except on weekends."

Kelly's gaze was hard. "And so it begins," he said. "Those cigars finally caught up to me."

"I told you that a long time ago."

"Yes. I know," replied Kelly.

The treatment went well, except that he had some difficulty swallowing after three weeks. He also lost weight.

"I found a new drink for people who have radiation therapy to their throat," said Kelly. "In the interests of advancing medicine, I thought I'd share it with you."

"What's that?" asked Matt.

"I used to drink scotch and water. But it burns my throat when I drink it now. I've switched to scotch and milk and it works great. The milk lines your throat when you swallow the whiskey."

"It would be better if you didn't drink at all. I hope you're not still smoking those cigars."

"I refuse to answer that question on the grounds that it might incriminate me."

"You sound just like a lawyer," said Matt.

Don Kelly continued his busy political agenda.

Finally, fourteen months later, he came in with more soreness in his throat and difficulty swallowing. A cinefluoroscopy was done. In this test the patient swallows radiopaque barium and, as he swallows, a movie is made of the swallowing mechanism. Abnormalities in the throat can be detected in this way. Sure enough, he had a cancer now involving part of the voice box and back of his throat.

"You have a fairly large cancer involving your voice box and esophagus," said Matt.

"What are my choices? Or do I have any?"

"You've had extensive radiation, so you can't have that any more. You can have chemotherapy but unfortunately, we don't have any drugs that work well with this type of cancer. You can have radical surgery with removal of the voice box and esophagus. You wouldn't be able to swallow or speak normally after that operation but you might live longer. Or periodically, I can take you into the operating room and with a hot cautery knife remove the bulk of the tumor so you can swallow. The last option, of course, is to do nothing. If you want a second opinion, we can also arrange that."

"I'll think about it."

The next afternoon, Matt received a call from one of Mr. Kelly's daughters.

"We'd like you to meet with the members of our family to discuss Dad's problem. We'd like you to cancel your office hours today, and we'll pay you for any money you lose."

"I can't do that. I've got twenty patients scheduled to see me. However, I take Thursday afternoons off. I could meet with you then."

"I'm sure that will be all right," replied the daughter.

On Thursday afternoon, the entire entourage of the Kelly family came into Matt's office. He briefly outlined Mr. Kelly's condition to the family members.

Frank Kelly, the eldest son, spoke up first. "I want my father to have the best care available. I want him to go to Massachusetts General Hospital in Boston."

"That's fine. I'll have to make some phone calls first, and he'll have to go by ambulance. We'll send him up to Boston by the end of the week if you like."

"No," said a son-in-law. "I want my father-in-law to go to the best cancer center in the world, Memorial Sloan Kettering in New York City."

"That's OK, too. I trained there and I'm sure we can get someone to see him. He'll also have to go by ambulance to New York City."

"No. We're not going to do anything until we talk with your father," said Mrs. Kelly. "One of you girls can go with me and Dr. Kendall, and we'll see what Dad wants to do."

The controversy, as to where he was to go for another opinion, was presented to Mr. Kelly.

"I don't need another opinion! I've put my trust in Dr. Kendall's hands for four years and I'm still alive. He's taken good care of me. As for those two who want me to go in an ambulance to New York City or Boston, forget it. I can still make my own decisions."

"I could arrange a phone consultation with some of the leading head and neck surgeons around the country. You wouldn't have to go anywhere," said Matt. "If you'd like I'll set it up."

"If it would make the family happy, do it. I'm staying put right here in this hospital. I like Whitestone Hospital!"

The next week, copies of Mr. Kelly's records were sent to the top head and neck cancer specialists around the country. A phone conference with Boston, New York City, Chicago, Houston, and Mexico City took place. One of Mr. Kelly's sons-in-law, a lawyer, listened to the entire phone conversation.

Dr. Kendall told each doctor on the phone to present their opinion and that the phone conference would be recorded for review.

Most felt that Mr. Kelly had too large a tumor to benefit from chemotherapy. The consultants thought there was very little to offer in his case, since he had multicentric cancer in various areas of the oral cavity. He would probably get other areas of involvement in the future.

Since Mr. Kelly didn't want radical surgery and was willing to accept the consequences, the consensus was to debulk the tumor in the oral cavity periodically and hope for the best.

The next day, Matt met with the patient's son-in-law.

"That was some phone conference," he replied. "They all seemed to know and respect you. I feel a lot better and the rest of the family does, too. We'll support your recommendation completely."

The entire phone consultation was then discussed with Mr. Kelly, his wife, and daughter. Kelly definitely did not want radical surgery and elected to come into the hospital periodically to have the bulk of the tumor removed. He said he'd take his chances.

"I've had a full, enjoyable and productive life. I'm ready to meet my maker," he said.

During this time, Watergate had become a national scandal, and Nixon was resigning the presidency. Kelly was getting over a hundred phone calls a day from around the country. Matt overheard many of these conversations. One call was from Senator "Scoop" Jackson from the West Coast.

"He's one of our greatest senators," said Kelly. "He'd make a great president."

Later that week, Mr. Kelly called Matt's office and said he wanted to speak to him about an urgent matter. Matt got on the phone.

"You've got to fire that old private duty nurse I have," Kelly said. "I can't tolerate her. She's always primping the bed, driving me nuts. She told me not to drink my scotch and milk that I've got here. Get rid of her!"

"It's not that easy. The nursing service assigns private duty nurses to the patients. She's one of our senior nurses. You're going to get me into hot water."

"I hired her, I can fire her," said Kelly. "I don't want her! Do anything to get her out of here. If I had an emergency, she wouldn't know what to do. All she does is primp up the pillows and straighten the sheets. Who the hell needs her?"

Kelly was adamant, so Matt went to the nursing service office and told the supervisor that Mr. Kelly wanted a younger, more alert nurse taking care of him.

"You're going to have to fire her, Dr. Kendall," said the nursing supervisor. "She may submit a grievance against you."

"Swell, I'm back in the middle," said Matt.

The next afternoon, he went over to see Mr. Kelly. In Matt's presence, Kelly told the nurse she was fired. She was quite upset.

"We'll talk about it in the hall," Matt said to her, and when they were alone in the corridor, she lost her temper.

"He can't do that to me! I'm expecting a bonus when he dies."

"Well, you're off the case. You can talk to Mr. Kelly some more if you want. He's the boss. But I wouldn't bitch about losing your bonus just because he persists in living."

She went in to see him and he repeated that she was fired. "I don't like the way you do your nursing," he said. He offered her one month's severance pay. She took the check and was crying as she left the room.

The next afternoon, there was a good-looking, 30-year-old blond divorced nurse assigned to the case, and the sparkle was back in Mr. Kelly's eyes.

"Now that's what I call a good nurse," he said.

The longer Dr. Kendall took care of Donald Kelly the more he respected him. Often, when he went in to see him, Mr. Kelly was obviously suffering but he rarely complained. He still had a keen mind and knew not only how to work with politicians, but how to get them to work together.

One day, Deane Allen, who was later made the Republican National Chairman, came to see Kelly in the hospital.

Dr. Kendall walked into Mr. Kelly's private room when Mr. Allen was visiting. When Allen left, Matt said, "He's from the opposing side. I can't believe how well you two get along."

Mr. Kelly thought for a minute and then replied. "We respect each other. We're good friends. He's been on the winning side and the losing side and I've been on the winning side and the losing side. The two-party system is the strength of this country. We both recognize that sometimes it's better to lose than to win. You can get a demagogue or unrecognized dictator who gets to control this country, so both of us try to do what we think is best for our country first. Then we consider what's best for our party.

"Take this thing with Nixon and Watergate. His biggest mistake was that he didn't destroy the tapes. Mr. Nixon knew a lot about foreign policy but his head was too big. He was on an ego trip."

Matt listened attentively as Kelly continued.

"Someday a woman will be vice president. The woman governor of Connecticut could fill that bill. And there's a black woman representative in Texas who could also do the job. It probably will be a black woman before a black man. You see, politically she would attract the women's vote and, because she's black, she would attract the black male vote."

"What do you think will be this country's biggest problem in the future?" asked Matt.

"Probably chaos within the country that will lead to destruction of what our constitution stands for."

"From within?" asked Matt. "You don't think Communism poses a threat?"

"Not at all," said Kelly. "If we continue to be innovative and productive in this country and defend our borders without destroying our economy, I don't believe we have anything to fear from the outside. What we do have to worry about most is our own leadership on both sides of the aisle. In centuries past, many empires have risen and fallen. The Roman Empire, for example. Incidentally, have you read the *Decline and Fall of the Roman Empire?*"

"By Gibbon?" asked Matt. "No, I have not."

"It's a tome," said Mr. Kelly. "Something like seventeen volumes. But I have. Every politician should. It tells you how an empire was destroyed by greed. In order to be reelected, the judges and the magistrates gave away everything they had. They created a gigantic welfare state. Pretty soon there were more people receiving the perks than there were workers to pay for them and the empire collapsed.

"We've had some great presidents in this country. I particularly liked Jefferson, Lincoln, and John Kennedy. If Kennedy had lived, he would have been one of the greatest. I was very fond of John Kennedy. It was a tragedy beyond belief when he was shot. In fact, I often wonder whether they protect our presidents enough. Oh, Harry Truman would be included in that list also. There's a man who was being shot at in the Blair House and he was sticking his head up to see what all the commotion was about. Harry Truman had to make some of the most crucial decisions in the history of this country and he made the right ones."

"Well, I'm alive because he dropped the atomic bomb," said Matt. "Your family seems to be very involved in politics. Do you have a favorite?"

"My smartest politician is my daughter. I'm very proud of her. She'll be in Congress someday. Hell, she could even be president!"

Later that week, at five o'clock, Matt went up to the Gold Coast section of the hospital to see Kelly. When he walked in, Kelly was stretched out on his stomach and the nurse was giving him a back-rub.

"Now you can see why I'm happy," said Mr. Kelly. "This gal is terrific. She really knows how to give a good Swedish massage."

Mr. Kelly's relationship with his new nurse grew as the days went on. Then one day, Matt received a phone call from Mr. Kelly's wife, Joan.

"Dr. Kendall, this is Joan Kelly. You know that Mr. Kelly will be going to the inauguration of President Ford down in Washington, DC. My husband, who is a past Chairman of the National Democratic Party, is expected to attend."

"I understand," said Matt.

"Well, he told me that you advised him to take Marilyn, that blonde nurse, with him to Washington, in case he had any trouble."

"I never told him that, but it might be a good idea."

"I thought so," said Joan. "She's going to get fired and this time I'll do the firing."

"Thanks a lot. Your family is really creating a great relationship for me with the nursing service."

17

MATT'S FATHER —"Pop" to his children—was a small, thin, wiry man, and toughened from working on construction for many years. He was also very opinionated and difficult to talk to. To his children, he was a strict disciplinarian, and even after he fell through the floor of a construction job and underwent skull surgery, he continued in life with his full mental capacities.

His pride and joy and symbol of his independence was his car, a Volkswagen Beetle. Around town he'd cruise, usually at a good clip, and would occasionally take unplanned trips. Pop had many escapades with the Beetle and they became more interesting as he approached 90 years of age. The aging process was taking its toll.

Shortly after his ninetieth birthday, he took his Beetle out for a spin and got pulled over by a state trooper. As the trooper walked up to the Beetle, Pop began to sweat.

"Let me see your registration please."

"What's that?" asked Pop. He was slightly hard of hearing.

"Your car registration, sir," said the officer.

"Oh yes." The elderly man's hands were shaking. He reached toward the glove compartment and pulled out a case that had, written in large letters across the top, "Car registration."

Pop's eyesight wasn't too good. He wore thick glasses, and the big letters on the leather case helped. It had been put there by his sons, one a lawyer and judge and the other a doctor.

"How long have you been driving?" asked the officer, realizing he was dealing with an elderly man.

Pop thought about the question. He had owned a Packard sedan back in 1927 that did about 25 m.p.h. Cars were one of his hobbies. He loved to tinker with the motors. Should he tell him he'd been driving a car for more than 60 years?

"Well?" repeated the officer. "How long have you been driving?"

"Quite a while," Pop replied, sheepishly.

"Do you realize that you were driving on the wrong side of the road?"

How should I answer that one? thought Pop. I thought I was driving on the right side of the road. He remembered seeing some cars driving across the road with brakes screeching. He had nearly hit three or four cars head on and couldn't understand what was going on. He was a little confused.

"Are you sure I was driving on the wrong side of the road?"

"Yes. I'm sure," said the officer.

Pop thought for a minute. When he drove out of the gas station, he thought the way he was supposed to go looked a little unfamiliar. Instead of turning right he had turned left and almost got hit by a speeding car. He remembered calling out to the driver, "You crazy jackass. Why don't you learn how to drive!"

"You've got me confused, officer. What can I say?"

"Let me have your registration please."

Pop handed the leather case over to the officer.

"You stay in your car while I check on your registration. I have to call in on my radio."

Pop sat in his Volkswagen. He cupped his face in his hands. He was dejected. What have I done? he thought. How can I get out of this one?

The officer got into his cruiser and picked up the mike.

"Connie, I need to have verification on a Volkswagen registration driven by an elderly male, Connecticut citizen. The license plate is ERG 1. Who do you have the car registered to?" There was a lengthy pause.

"To a Mr. Kendall," said Connie.

"What's the date of birth?" asked the officer.

"It's hard to read," said Connie. "I think it says 1895."

"Brother, this guy's 91 years old and still driving a car. That name's familiar to me," said the officer.

"It should be," said Connie. "One of his sons is a superior court judge and his other son is a prominent surgeon at Whitestone Hospital."

"Well, I better get on the phone with one of his sons. This guy was driving on the wrong side of the road. Luckily, no one got hurt. But three or four cars ended up in the ditch and he kept coming straight at me until he saw my flashing lights. I'll call the judge. Where can I locate him?"

"He's usually sitting in session in the Superior Courthouse," said Connie. "You might have trouble getting to him. Why don't you try the doctor's office? His office is right next to Whitestone Hospital."

"Do you have his phone number?"

"I can look it up for you."

The officer got Dr. Kendall's phone number and called his office. Judy picked up the phone. "Dr. Kendall's office, may I help you?"

"Yes," said Trooper Donovan. "I'd like to talk to the doctor if possible. His father almost got into an auto accident about an hour ago. He almost ran into me."

"I'll get the doctor for you. Hold on please," said Judy.

"Dr. Kendall, your father is in trouble again. He almost hit a state trooper's car."

"You've got to be kidding."

"The trooper's on the phone."

Matt punched line one. "Dr. Kendall speaking."

"Dr. Kendall, this is Officer Donovan. Your father almost hit my car head on going against the traffic."

"Did he hurt anyone? Is he all right?" asked Matt.

"No. He's fine. But he's a little depressed about my calling you."

"He ought to be," said Matt, knowing the significance of the call. Pop had said once the keys to his car were taken away from him he'd rather be dead. His car was his greatest liberty, his sign of freedom.

"What do you want me to do?" asked Matt. "I'm tied up right now and I'm going into emergency surgery in a few minutes. I'll call my brother and have him help straighten this mess out."

"Your father doesn't want your brother to be called. He really shouldn't be driving, you know," said the state trooper.

"I agree. We've been trying to tell him that for a long time. I'll call my brother and have him call you right back."

He called his brother, Judge Mark Kendall. Luckily he was in his chambers.

"Mark, this is Matt. Pop got into trouble with that Volkswagen again."

"What happened?"

"He almost hit a state trooper, head on."

"That's great! Did he get hurt?"

"No."

"Did he hurt anybody?"

"No."

"Are you free to pick him up?"

"No. It's your turn. I drove up to Maine to pick him up the last time. He was all the way to Maine when we got that call from the pharmacist in Portland. He's only just east of the river this time."

"OK, I'll handle it," said the judge. "I'll declare a recess. Let me have the phone number. You know what this means, don't you? Pop is going to get depressed as hell when we take his car keys away."

"I know, but luckily he isn't going to be put in jail for hitting a state trooper head on. That, at least, is something to be thankful for."

The two sons decided to talk to Pop together and tell him why he could no longer drive. The older son, Mark, did the talking.

"Pop, you almost killed a cop driving against the traffic. We can't let you drive anymore. We're taking away the keys to your Volkswagen Beetle."

There were tears in Pop's eyes and he was visibly shaken. He finally spoke to his sons.

"You know what this is going to do to me. It's going to kill me. My freedom will be gone."

After that meeting, Pop's personality changed completely. He became a shell of his past. The gleam in his eyes went and he lost interest in eating. He lost weight and he became sloppy with his dress. A few months later, he had a massive stroke and died in his sleep.

Pop was fortunate that he had his mental capacities right up to the age of 90. Many times that does not happen. Any surgeon who does major surgery will eventually have a patient who remains in a vegetative state.

Once a patient's mental capacity has been seriously affected by an illness, it is too late to decide how much effort should be made by the medical staff to prolong that individual's life. It becomes ever clearer that this decision should be made before any extensive surgery.

Living wills allow the wishes of the patient to be implemented, if and when they develop a terminal illness. Most state legislatures have laws concerning living wills, and recently the Supreme Court helped define just treatment of the incompetent patient when it ruled on the case of Nancy Cruzan—a young girl who was kept alive for a very long period of time after she was brain dead.

Medicine has made tremendous advances in patient care during the past 30 years. New equipment can prolong life, though its use may be counter to the wishes of the patient. Moral and ethical problems surrounding the patient care have led to legal confrontations.

There are some medical practitioners who agree with the Hippocratic Oath, which states that life should be preserved and sustained by all available means and that no doctor should assist in hastening the demise of the patient. Other practitioners have recently challenged that concept and the courts are still involved in sorting through the legalities and ethics of that dilemma.

As the doctor's ability to use life-sustaining measures have improved, there has been a commensurate challenge to determine the purpose of it. The pain and suffering some diseases bring are overwhelming, and the cost of maintaining life becomes prohibitive.

After being in surgical practice for several years, Matt was confronted with the management and care of a patient with terminal cancer.

The patient was a successful insurance executive who was a heavy smoker. He had emphysema of the lungs and bladder cancer, necessitating a resection of his bladder and the creation of a new bladder out of the small bowel. He wore a bag to collect his urine on the right side of his abdominal wall.

Dr. Kendall had performed the operation. The patient did well for three years, although he continued to be a chain smoker. He was encouraged to stop but refused to, claiming it was his only remaining pleasure in life.

Finally, because of his progressive shortness of breath, he had to carry a portable oxygen tank. An x-ray was taken after he developed increasing respiratory trouble and sure enough, a large mass had developed in his lung. A biopsy diagnosed lung cancer, and further studies revealed that he was inoperable because many other areas of his body were involved with cancer. He had developed a second primary cancer.

It was decided that x-ray treatment would not help because it would damage the remaining good lung surface and only compound his breathing problem. Matt had a medical oncologist make a brief attempt to use chemotherapy, but the patient could not take the toxic side effects and refused to continue.

The patient was eventually relegated to Dr. Kendall's care as a patient in the hospital because he had performed the cystectomy and ileal conduit for his bladder.

The patient required continuous oxygen, frequent morphine shots for pain, and he had the blue cast of cyanosis. It was impossible for the patient to remain outside the oxygen tent. He was particularly demanding, requiring constant nursing care.

When Matt went on vacation he usually got one of the senior surgeons to cover him. Usually he preferred Jack Diamond, the Chief of Surgery.

"Jack, there are three surgical cases for you to watch for me while I'm away," he said before leaving.

"Give me the list and I'll take care of them," Jack replied. "Anything I should know about them?"

"Not really, except for the man who's on the urology floor. He's an insurance executive with bladder and lung cancer. He's inoperable and he's been dying for the past six months with emphysema, bladder cancer, and lung cancer."

"Why doesn't he die?"

"He's too mean," said Matt. "The nurses all hate him. He requires constant care. He's excessively demanding; some of them would dance if he'd pass on. He's always cyanotic and requires continuous oxygen in the O_2 tent. He's mentally out of it 90 percent of the time."

"Why don't you shut it off and just let him die?"

"I'd like to and I'm sure he'd like to have it shut off, but his son's a lawyer and monitors his care."

"Those goddamn lawyers are always screwing things up," Jack replied. "They're the biggest babies when they get sick. But listen, I'll take care of your cases. Have a good vacation. You going to play golf?"

"Yes. And I hope to do some fishing too."

"Well, you deserve it. Cancer patients are the toughest. That's why I'm a general surgeon."

Matt went on his vacation with his wife and children for two weeks in Naples, played golf, fished, and decompressed from the world of surgery.

When he got back from vacation, he went to the urology floor to see his terminally ill patient. There was another patient in the room.

"What happened to Mr. Hill?" he asked the head nurse.

"He was found dead in bed a week ago."

"Did they do an autopsy to check on the cause?"

"No. They knew he had lung and bladder cancer and emphysema. Enough to kill anybody. He suffered for so long, it's a blessing he died."

When Matt saw Jack he asked, "Any problems while I was gone?"

"Not really."

"What happened to Mr. Hill?"

Jack stepped closer. "While you were away, I had to come into the hospital one evening to do an appendix. I dropped by to see Mr. Morrison, the insurance executive in the bed next to Hill's. I tripped over the cord for the O_2 getting pumped into his tent. I didn't realize what happened. The nurses tell me he died quietly in his sleep."

Matt stared at Diamond. "You didn't realize what happened?"

"He's in the arms of God, Matt. Let it be."

Matt held his gaze on the Chief, gauging him. Finally he said, "Thanks for covering for me when I was gone."

"It was my pleasure," said Diamond. The two men looked at each other. Matt knew something had passed between them and he knew there was a tacit agreement that what happened was for the best.

That night, Matt lay in bed thinking. He knew that Hill's body had been ravaged by cancer. The man's lungs and bladder were riddled. Hill was miserable, physically miserable. His personality was a reflection of his physical state. What troubled Matt was not what Jack had done. It was a relief. Matt knew Diamond, and he would never be clumsy enough to trip over something as vital as the cord to a life support unit.

So there it was. He would do nothing. If left within him the lingering disquiet of a moral dilemma unsolved. Euthanasia.

The following week, he was asked to see one of the Broadway stars of the show "The Solid Gold Cadillac." Her medical history was quite interesting. After a long run, the show was taken on the road. Then, while in Chicago, she developed unexplained hoarseness and her understudy had to take her part. An ENT professor from Chicago had looked in her throat and couldn't find anything wrong.

With medication she did somewhat better but in Boston she regressed. She had increasing hoarseness. She was seen at Mass. Eye and Ear and another doctor looked in her throat and told her to stop smoking. She was told to rest her voice, so she left the troupe and went home to Pomfret, Connecticut. But her condition persisted and she ended up in the office of an ENT doctor at Whitestone Hospital who knew Matt. He referred the patient to him.

"I'd like to do a direct laryngoscopy to look at your throat," said Matt. "I know you've had it done before but I might see something that the others missed."

"Well, I can't go on like this," said the star. "Hoarseness is not tolerable on the stage. I stopped smoking, but that hasn't helped. Resting hasn't improved it either. How soon can you do it?"

"We'll admit you and do it tomorrow."

"Fine. Get me a private room with a bath."

The next day, she was taken to the operating room and her throat was anesthetized with a local anesthetic.

Matt gently inserted a Jakoscope laryngoscope with fiberoptic lights and looked at the vocal chords. They showed some damage from the persistent smoking but there was no tumor. He then looked in the pyriform fossa on both sides of the voice box and there was a gray haziness on the mucus membranes. He decided to do some biopsies, taking tissue with cutting forceps and placing it in a preservative so it could be stained and looked at under the microscope. The pathologists checked it, and found it was a cancer.

The next day, Matt told her the bad news.

"I'm sorry to tell you this, but we've found your trouble. You have a squamous cell cancer of the right hypopharynx." Matt braced himself for hysterics, tears, and then, in a while, silence.

Her reply was unexpected. "Thank goodness," she said. "I knew those filthy cigarettes would catch up to me someday. Now, by golly, I know what's wrong. Well, young man, what should we do about it?"

"You have three choices. The first is radical surgery that would remove the tumor with your voicebox. The second is radiation therapy that would preserve your voicebox but you would continue to have hoarseness. Or both; surgery followed by radiation therapy. Oh, there's a fourth. You could do nothing."

"Well," she said briskly, "that finishes my career on Broadway. I'm going to have to think about this. I live in New York City. Can I have radiation treatment down there if I want to?"

"Of course. If that's what you choose, I'll help arrange it."

The actress called him three days later. "I've decided to have radiation treatment and take my chances. My doctor on Park Avenue is going to set up the treatment. He's an internist and works at Sloan Kettering. He says he remembers you as a resident."

Matt thought about that Broadway star—she was made of iron. He'd rarely seen anyone so practical and decisive about her life.

Three years later, she returned, having developed a recurrence of her throat cancer that was obstructing her airway. They consulted, and reviewed her options. She had Matt do a total laryngectomy and neck dissection, completely removing her voicebox. Her postoperative recovery at Whitestone was smooth except for one problem. Every day she'd read the Wall Street Journal and have her private nurse call her broker in New York. She bought and sold as much as $50,000 worth of stock a day, even though she was heavily medicated.

Matt finally called her lawyer in New York and told him about it.

"Doctor, I wouldn't worry about it. She's worth millions. Let her have her fun."

Matt thought about that for a moment, and realized he didn't want to be liable for stock losses due to decisions made under medication. "Do me a favor and put your statement in writing," he said.

"I'll be glad to," he replied.

Three years later the Broadway star was back at Whitestone. This time she had diffuse recurrent cancer. She was having difficulty swallowing and had developed a second primary cancer in her lungs.

"Dr. Kendall, you've kept me alive for seven years and I'm grateful for that, but I'm ready to meet my maker. A month ago I had a long talk with my hotshot lawyer in New York and told him to write up a living will. You're a bargain, compared to him, by the way. But I wanted to pay his bill before I died and I told him I didn't want any tubes, or intravenous feedings, and just enough oxygen to keep me comfortable. I expect you to abide by my wishes also. It's all in this signed and notarized living will."

Matt accepted the legal paper and read it. "I respect your wishes and will carry them out," he said. Three weeks later she quietly died in her sleep.

Matt thought about the two cases; the terminal, embittered insurance executive, and the Broadway star. The insurance executive had been a small, mean man in agony, with little to live for in the way of family, love, and money. No one had visited him. He was alone in his final days. The star knew life to be rich, extravagant, daring, and filled with fame. Her admirers were many, her detractors confined to theater critics and jealous show biz people. In her last days, she showed only grace and strength in facing death. Mr. Hill clung desperately to a life that seemed only to provide moment-to-moment pain.

It raised interesting questions. Was the gift of life so profoundly powerful that one would cling to it through immense suffering? Could one choose beforehand how one would accept the inevitable? Matt had never really dwelled on death; all his work and skill went toward preserving life.

During the next 15 years more and more of his patients ended up in the intensive care unit. His major surgical cases had increased and he was being sent more difficult tumor cases. Many were elderly. He noticed the intensive care unit had increased in size, the nursing personnel had improved, and that most of the patients now had expensive monitoring equipment attached to them. The equipment was electronically controlled with sensors so the pulse, blood pressure, and oxygenation of the tissues were constantly monitored.

He also saw that not all of the patients in the unit were elderly people; there were several young patients who were motorcycle or auto accident victims, who were brain dead, but nothing else was wrong with them. Most of them were candidates for organ donations.

Oxygen tents had been done away with, and endotracheal tubes that extended into the lungs were either protruding from their noses or mouths, maintaining oxygenation of the tissues. The cost of having a patient in the intensive care unit had skyrocketed—it was over $2,000 a day and still rising.

New types of doctors ran the ICU. They were called intensivists and some had had training in large metropolitan centers to learn the best methods for caring for these extremely sick patients.

Man is an animal who, when you put him on his back for any length of time, will develop all sorts of complications. Pressure of the weight of the back on the hospital bed can lead to breakdown of tissues and special types of bed mattresses were developed to prevent permanent damage and bed sores. Bowel and kidney problems develop rapidly due to stasis, and coagulopathy can develop causing clots (emboli) that can migrate to vital organs.

For those patients with damaged kidneys who need dialysis, prolonged sophisticated feeding methods are used with permanent intravenous shunts. Sometimes openings in the stomach are used as feeding tubes. Scanning devices to determine heart muscle function after heart surgery and vascular angiography are other methods used to determine a patient's condition. All these methods require special monitoring and care, which explains to some degree the increased costs.

The right-to-die issue became personal when Dr. Kendall's secretary got him involved in the care of her mother. "She's in the ICU," said Judy.

"Dr. Rutstein doesn't tell me anything and I'm getting tired of bringing her in by ambulance every month or so. I'm trying to take care of two teenage daughters as well as my mother. My father's dead so I'm the one who has to make all the decisions."

"Tell me a little about your mother's history."

"She's seventy-two years old and an insulin-dependent diabetic who's had chronic obstructive pulmonary disease for years. She's a heavy smoker and she's had both carotid arteries in her neck operated on for obstructive disease. She's had several heart attacks and little strokes in the past and has had a pacemaker for two years. She's been in the intensive care unit five times this year and is usually there for four or five weeks at a time."

"Why don't you put her in a convalescent home?"

"I can't afford it and her insurance won't pay for it."

"Idiots! The insurance company must be paying a bigger chunk for that intensive care unit. You'd think it would be better for them to pay for convalescent home care than those hospital admissions. Does your mother want all those tubes and things used to help keep her alive?"

"No. She's told me many times that she's ready to die and she's miserable living the way she is."

"Have you told her doctor this?"

"Many times. So has my mother."

"What does he say?"

"He says his job is to keep people alive, not to help them die. He keeps telling me he took the Hippocratic Oath."

"That's a laugh. Isn't he the doctor that charges patients if they don't show up for appointments?"

"Yes, he's done that to my mother, too."

"When we finish up in the office today I'll go over to the hospital with you and see your mother."

When they got to the intensive care unit, Judy's mother had an endotracheal tube in her throat, was on a respirator, and was still having difficulty breathing. She had fluid in both lungs and had a Foley catheter in place to measure her urine output. Her hands were tied down so she couldn't pull the tubes out. She had already pulled them out several times. She was heavily sedated.

Dr. Kendall talked to the resident in the medical intensive care unit. "Dr. Hewett, I wonder if you'd tell me about my secretary's mother in bed eight."

"Well, she's got multisystem problems—heart, lungs, kidneys, liver—you name it. She's tough to take care of because she pulls her endotracheal tube out all the time. She's pulled it out ten times on this admission. Anesthesia is getting tired of putting it back in."

"Is she ever conscious?"

"She's not too bad right now," he said. "Pinch her and she'll open her eyes."

Judy went over and touched her mother and she opened her eyes and squeezed her daughter's hand.

"Dr. Kendall came over to see you," said Judy. "I want you to answer his questions. He's here to help. He cares."

"How do you feel?" asked Matt.

She made a bad face.

"Judy told me you don't want all these tubes in. Is that right?"

She nodded her head. There were tears in her eyes and in her daughter's eyes as they looked at each other.

The next day Dr. Kendall talked to her mother's doctor. "My secretary doesn't want her mother to have all those tubes in. Can't you do something about it?"

"Sorry, I don't believe in pulling the plug. I also don't want to be sued. As long as the patient can still open her eyes her brain is still functioning as far as I'm concerned. She has excellent major medical coverage and there's no reason why the insurance won't continue to pay her bills."

After talking to Dr. Rutstein, Matt and Judy sat down and wrote a letter stating that all life-sustaining measures be stopped and that nature must be allowed to take its course. A lawyer reviewed the letter and it was notarized and signed by Judy before being sent to the doctor with a copy filed in the hospital chart.

Dr. Rutstein ignored the letter. He gave orders for her endotracheal tube to be replaced every time she pulled it out. The patient was also given a blood transfusion (for reasons that were never explained) after the letter was put in her file. Judy didn't know about the transfusion until she received the bill from the hospital. Finally, Judy threatened to sue the doctor if he prolonged her mother's agony and suffering.

That worked. Her mother was eventually transferred to a convalescent home and five days after arriving, she died quietly in her sleep.

But her death was only the beginning of more hardship. Judy received her mother's bill from the hospital, which included a $5,000 charge from the anesthesia department for reinsertion of her endotracheal tube 25 times during the last hospital admission. The hospital bill alone was over $4,000 a day for seven weeks.

Dr. Rutstein sent a bill for $5,000 for his care, even though he was on vacation for three weeks while the patient was in the hospital. The medical resident in the intensive care unit wrote most of the orders on the chart.

"I'd like to put Dr. Rutstein out of business," said Judy. "He'd make a better snake-oil salesman than a doctor!"

Matt advised her to write a letter to the County Medical Society regarding Dr. Rutstein and his actions, but she decided to try to forget the situation and be consoled with the fact that her mother was no longer being kept alive against her wishes and was no longer suffering.

18

MATT'S PRACTICE was flourishing—he had more than enough surgery to do. He was referred difficult cancer cases from around the state and he took pride in doing a good job. He received the most important reward that a good surgeon can get—most of his patients got well. His extra training at Memorial Sloan Kettering Cancer Center in New York had given him an intellectual independence that was reflected in his results. A strong bond was established between himself and his patients and more and more of his referrals came directly from them.

It was ironic when he looked back and thought of that day when he was applying for surgical privileges to the chief of surgery at Whitestone Hospital, and was told that he would not be allowed to work in the ER to build up his practice. What a shame! The old-boy method of control had not succeeded.

Dramatic changes were developing in the ER at Whitestone Hospital—more and more poor were using the emergency room as their family doctor and as a result the total volume of patients was bogging down the efficiency of the ER.

The hospital had hired full-time physicians to improve its efficiency but it wasn't working.

Matt's own family had grown. Betsy was 17 years old and looking over prospective colleges. Mike was 15 years old, playing football and hockey for his high school team. Susan was 11 years old, and Karen, the youngest, was 7 years old.

They were all bright youngsters, all did well in their classes. Each was an individualist trying to achieve excellence. Nancy was a compassionate mother—constantly reading to them and nurturing their interests. She encouraged them to try to acquire the habit of reading and to enjoy it.

They all had specific activities that required her time and she willingly gave it to them. She loved them dearly and they loved her.

Betsy had struggled in elementary school, getting poor grades because it wasn't recognized that she needed glasses. Matt and Nancy had Betsy's eyes examined by an excellent ophthalmologist when she was in the second grade and he had reassured them that her eyes were perfect.

One day, when Betsy was in the third grade, Matt came home from work and saw her sitting right in front of the television set so he spoke to her.

"Don't sit so close to the TV set, Betsy."

"That's the only way I can see the picture, Daddy," she replied.

That did it! Matt took her to one of the senior ophthalmologists at the hospital who examined her and said she needed glasses. She was 20/80 in one eye and 20/60 in the other.

The day she came home from school after wearing her new glasses for the first time she brought tears to Nancy and Matt's eyes when she said, "I can see the blackboard now, Daddy."

Betsy seemed to be always running to catch up after that. However, she finally did catch up in her junior and senior year of high school, getting on the honor roll and being accepted to a great college in Pennsylvania.

Mike was active in sports and did well with his schoolwork. Every now and then, Matt would work on Mike, trying to get him to think about becoming a doctor. He didn't seem to be too interested. His comment was, "We don't see you that much, Dad. You seem to be working night and day. I'm not sure I want that kind of lifestyle."

Matt got the message but he didn't change his ways. All he thought about was the college tuition costs for four bright youngsters.

Susan was the easygoing daughter—as sweet and gentle as a girl could be. She was never in a hurry about anything. She was pretty and lots of boys were willing to carry her books for her. However, her sedate manners could fool you. She could really throw a curve ball at her family if she wanted to and did so on one occasion.

In junior high school, one of Susan's classmates brought a pack of cigarettes into school. A small group of girls knew about the cigarettes and made some plans. They wanted to be just like the grownups, smoking cigarettes and looking sophisticated.

In their activity class they would raise their hand and ask to be excused to go to the bathroom. There was a rule at school that there was to be no smoking in the bathrooms. Susan was number seven on the list to try the cigarettes and by this time the homeroom teacher suspected that something was going on outside her classroom. In the girls' bathroom, it was like an Indian pow-wow meeting of the chiefs with smoke rings coming out of the doors.

Susan was shocked when she saw her teacher peering over the top edge of the stall as she puffed on a cigarette while sitting on the throne. It was the shock of her young life! She had to go in to see the principal and was given a note to take home to her parents.

Matt was given the note by Nancy as they all sat at the dinner table.

Matt's comment after reading the note was not appropriate in retrospect and he later felt sorry about making it.

"Susan, how could you do this to your Dad? I'm supposed to be a cancer specialist discouraging smoking and my daughter gets caught smoking cigarettes in the lavatory in junior high school. You should be ashamed of yourself!"

That remark was good for crying and a loud wail from Susan and a fast blast at Matt from Nancy.

"How could you make a remark like that to your daughter?" she said. "You ought to be ashamed of yourself. I suppose you never did anything foolish when you were a boy."

Karen, the youngest, got an overdose of everything from Nancy and Matt. Not only was she extremely intelligent, she was a tremendous individualist. In many ways she was their pride and joy.

"She reminds me of you," said Nancy. "She's going to beat the world someday!"

Matt eventually believed this and got an early indication of her potential when she was ten years old.

Matt bought and read the *New York Times* at his office daily. When his work day was done, he would bring it home to finish reading some of the articles he was interested in.

One day, he forgot to bring the paper home. His daughter Karen came up to him after dinner with tears in her eyes and her lower lip stuck out a mile long. She said, "Daddy, you didn't bring the *New York Times* home."

"What's that got to do with the price of eggs?" replied Matt. "Why do you want the *New York Times*?"

"I read the editorial page and pick out the words that I don't understand and look them up in the dictionary."

"Is that true, Nancy?" asked Matt.

"I guess it is because I see her looking at that paper quite a bit."

"Well, I'll be damned," replied Matt. "Karen, that will be the last time your Daddy forgets to bring the *New York Times* home."

Karen eventually went on to graduate as valedictorian of her class in high school.

As Matt's surgical practice grew, he started to get up earlier in the morning in order to see all his patients prior to surgery. He would have a light breakfast in the hospital cafeteria so that he could talk to the surgical residents about his patients. The Inner Sanctum Brain Trust invited him to become a regular member of their elite group. The resident doctors now had an additional title for the group—the Brahmin Super Peer Review Society. It was evident that no matter what they were called, all were successful in their medical specialties and were considered intellectuals with contrasting views. They came from varied socioeconomic and geographic backgrounds.

Criticism and controversy were common during the morning conversations. Most of the members of the Brain Trust were active in hospital politics at one time or another and served on various committees. Some were chairmen, and a few had gained recognition outside the local communities and served on committees in national or international medical societies.

"I've noticed that Bill Jones, the general practitioner in Bloomfield, doesn't come into the hospital anymore," said Bill Milstein.

"That's right," said Andrews. "He's pissed off at the increased cost of his malpractice insurance. He's mad at the lawyers and the insurance companies and now he refers all his difficult cases to hospital-based specialists to get the difficult cases off his back. He's convinced the lawyers and the insurance companies are in cahoots to grab some of the income the doctors are making. You should hear him—he says they're a mutual admiration society that's economically beneficial to themselves."

"But the populace gets hurt, right?" suggested Milstein.

"That's right," said Steve Walters. "The more the doctors have to pay for malpractice, the more the cost of health care goes up. If you pay one-hundred thousand dollars for malpractice insurance, you have to raise your fees or quit. Ultimately, the patient suffers."

"It's getting worse, isn't it?" suggested Dr. Alford.

"Dr. Jones told me he may go bare and not carry any malpractice insurance at all," said Andrews. "He's going to put all his assets in his wife's name."

"What happens when she runs off with a young gigolo?" asked Dr. Alford.

"I'd blow her brains out," said Milstein.

Walters, the young oncologist, cut through the chuckling, "Dr. Arnold, out in Ellington, recently got sued for delay in treatment on a colon case. He missed a rectal cancer because he didn't put his finger up a patient's ass. The patient thought he had hemorrhoids and was told to use Preparation H, which he did for three years. That case was just settled out of court for half a million bucks. He quit practice. He didn't have enough insurance to cover it. It's ironic. He's on the other side now. He took a full-time job with an insurance company."

"How many of you guys have been sued?" asked Bill Burns.

Three of the doctors seated at the table raised their hands.

"Every good doctor gets sued at least once," said Alford.

"Exactly," said Matt. "You have to take a risk sometimes to save a patient's life. In the operating room, one little slip of the knife and you can have a dead patient. With our population aging, the body's tissues sometimes aren't healthy or repairable, so when you operate on an alcoholic or a heavy smoker you're working against the odds. And they're the patients who sue you."

"Malpractice insurance will destroy medicine," said Burns. "The applications to law school have tripled and the applications to medical school have gone down. Why spend fifteen years of your life getting your medical education and go into the hole financially when you can go to law school for just three years?"

"I agree," said Matt. "It's pathetic! When I started practice, doctors were looked at with reverence. Now, as a surgeon, I have to work for three months just to pay my malpractice insurance. Doctors have been knocked off the pedestal they used to enjoy alongside the clergy."

"Amen," said Andrews. "When the lawyers lost the big settlements from auto accidents and no-fault insurance came into being, they had to find another source of income. So they got into the malpractice business."

"How many of them get sued?" asked Steve Walters.

"Very few. And their malpractice rates are minimal compared to ours. It doesn't cost them anything to defend themselves," said Bill Milstein.

"The other day, I took care of one of our senior malpractice lawyers in this city," said Bill Burns. "He couldn't piss, right? So I put a Foley catheter in to drain his urine. I biopsied his prostate and it was cancer. He wanted me to sign a paper to guarantee his sex life after I removed his prostate. I refused. He walked all over New York City with a Foley catheter in, trying to get a urologist to guarantee his sex life after the operation. No one was stupid enough to do it. He finally came back.

" 'Doc, you've got to help me,' he said, 'I've got to get rid of this rubber tube between my legs. I'll do whatever you want me to. I can't stand it anymore.' I told him he'd have to sign a paper saying he wouldn't sue me if he ended up with a zero sex life. The lawyer shrugged his shoulders and said, 'It's zero now anyhow.' He signed the paper and I did the operation."

"After the operation, the lawyer came to me and said, 'You know Doc, when you can't piss, it's painful as hell. Pissing is one of the most underrated thrills there is. I'm forever grateful.' "

Mr. Snow, the CEO of the hospital spoke up: "There has to be some better way to compensate the patient when an accident or undesired result occurs. Some of the lawyers take fifty percent of the settlement—they're the ones making a killing."

"That's not the problem," said Andrews. "No one wants to get sued—that's why all those CT scans, ultrasounds and MRIs are being done. It costs billions of dollars to do many unnecessary tests. Malpractice insurance costs and defensive medicine testing costs just add to the prohibitive cost of health care."

19

MATT WAS SOUND ASLEEP when the phone rang at twelve midnight. It was a golfing buddy of his on the phone.

"Doc, this is Fred Hogan. I feel miserable. I had a few drinks at the club, went to bed two hours ago and just vomited. I'm sick as a dog!"

"You just drank too much."

"It's not what you're thinking, Doc. I turned on the light in the bathroom and the bowl was filled with bright red blood. I'm sweaty and I feel like I'm going to die."

Matt remembered Fred. He had been the club champ, usually kept himself in good condition, and wasn't a heavy drinker.

"Tell your wife to drive you to the emergency room at Whitestone Hospital immediately. I'll meet you there."

He got on the phone and called the hospital. He talked to the emergency room and the chief resident surgeon on call.

"There's a forty-nine-year-old guy coming into the ER with upper gastrointestinal bleeding. He's real sick. I want you to see him as soon as he gets there. Also, see if there are any gastroenterologists in the house so he can be scoped to find out where he's bleeding from."

"I just finished a case with Dr. Fineberg. He does endoscopy. Do you want me to ask him to see the patient?"

"Sure, that'll be great. If he looks real sick when he gets in there alert the operating room so they'll have personnel available if we need them."

"Yes, sir," replied the resident.

Matt got dressed and drove to the ER in the middle of the night.

The patient got to the emergency room before he did and was seen by the resident, who passed a tube into his stomach and noted brisk bleeding. An IV was placed in his arm, blood studies were drawn, and a central line—a large bore needle for fluid and blood replacement—was inserted in his neck.

Dr. Douglas took a history of the patient's illness.

He was a white, healthy male who was well until the evening of his admission. He had eaten a large meal and stated that he had had quite a few pops of whiskey before going to bed rather early in the evening. He felt somewhat nauseous before going to bed. Around midnight he got sick, and had quite a bit of severe retching. He felt somewhat better after this and went back to bed but was unable to sleep. His wife told him he had a horrible odor about him. He started to sweat, developed palpitations, and felt like he was going to vomit again. He got out of bed, turned the light on in the bathroom and vomited into the bowl. He almost passed out when he saw the bowl filled with bright red blood.

He then got on the phone and called Matt. When he saw him in the emergency room, he was pale, bright red blood was draining rapidly from the tube placed in his stomach, his pulse was rapid, and his blood pressure was dropping.

"We better take this guy to the intensive care unit and alert the blood bank that we have a patient with a massive bleed in the unit. We're going to need lots of blood.

"You'd better get that G.I. doctor and tell him we want him to put a tube into this guy's stomach to see where he's bleeding from. Page him, stat," said Dr. Kendall.

The head nurse called the page operator.

"Dr. Fineberg, Dr. Fineberg, wanted in the ICU stat!"

A quick history was taken from the patient's wife. Fred had no previous stomach symptoms that would suggest an ulcer. Nor was he an alcoholic, who might have esophageal varices, which are veins that dilate in the esophagus that goes from the mouth to the stomach. If you drink too much and get cirrhosis of the liver, these veins can rupture and bleed.

"What's up?" asked Fineberg.

"We've got a guy with a massive upper G.I. bleed with no past history of ulcer and he's not an alcoholic. He's really pouring out the blood."

"Do we have the laser set up?"

"It's all set, Dr. Fineberg," said the nurse.

Dr. Fineberg passed a large, flexible tube through the patient's mouth, slowly down the esophagus to the stomach. The stomach was washed out with a continuous flush of water to see its inner lining.

"Matt, it looks like he's got a Mallory Weiss Syndrome," said Fineberg. "From all that vomiting and retching, he's got a large laceration or tear at the distal esophagus and stomach. The blood is really pumping out."

Matt took a look down the scope. Two torn blood vessels could be seen bleeding profusely at the junction of the esophagus and stomach.

"Do you think you can stop that bleeding with the laser?"

"I'll give it a try. I think I can zap it."

A fine instrument within the scope was placed against the bleeding site and the area was zapped with the laser to coagulate the blood.

The patient continued to bleed.

Dr. Fineberg was having trouble getting the bleeding to stop, and large amounts of water were pumped into the stomach to get rid of the blood clots.

The blood and water were suctioned out as the gastroenterologist tried to see where the bleeding was coming from with the lighted lens at the end of the tube. An arterial pumper (blood vessel) continued to bleed profusely. The patient bled out his total blood volume (seven pints of blood) within an hour. An interarterial infusion of a medicine used to constrict blood vessels (Pitressin) was administered, but the bleeding continued.

Laser coagulation was attempted again. Two or three additional attempts were tried to no avail.

"Dr. Kendall, the blood bank called. They have only two units of blood left. They're running out."

"Damn it! Tell them to bring in some donors! Call the operating room and tell them we're bringing this guy up. We have to crack his belly."

The patient was taken on a stretcher to the operating room, his blood running out through the tube. Anesthesia put him to sleep and Matt made a large upper midline incision in the belly and entered the abdomen right over the anterior surface of the stomach.

He grabbed the upper part of the stomach with two large Babcock clamps. The stomach looked like a blood-filled football. Matt cut open the upper part of the stomach. He reached his hand into the stomach and a big basin full of large clots came out. Using a metal sucker he saw two large arterial blood vessels pumping away in the upper part of the stomach. The bleeding sites that Dr. Fineberg had coagulated were very close to the bleeding vessels but not close enough. Matt quickly oversewed the blood vessels with heavy silk arterial sutures and the bleeding stopped. He washed out the stomach with saline solution and closed the stomach and abdomen rapidly with running stitches.

As Matt stepped away from the table, the entire area soaked in blood, he looked down to see color returning to Fred's face. In the reflection of a stainless steel lamp, Matt caught his own reflection, pale and drawn at 4:30 A.M., and he thought, hell, Fred looks better than I do.

Dr. Kendall got unpredictable and challenging referrals from the ER at Whitestone Hospital.

On one occasion, he got a phone call from the ER, at 4:30 A.M. It was from Dr. Perkins, one of the chief surgical residents.

"Dr. Kendall, you can't believe the case we've got here in the emergency room. In fact, you have to see it, to believe it."

"What do you mean? Whatcha got?"

"We have a big problem here and we need your help. We have a truck driver who got drunk, hit a pole, was thrown out of his cab, and landed on a metal picket fence."

"Is he still alive?"

"Yes. He's still alive. They had to cut the picket fence out of the ground and bring it in with him. Part of the fence is still sticking in him."

"Why are you calling me?"

"Because the fence went right through his neck, above his larynx. Dr. Johnson told us to call you. He's a new plastic surgeon on our staff. He wants someone who knows the head and neck anatomy to help."

"I'll be right in. It sounds like he ought to be taken to the OR right away and have a tracheostomy tube put in, with a cuff on it."

"We've already alerted the OR. When you get here, he'll be there."

Twenty minutes later, Matt arrived on the operating room floor. The OR supervisor met him at the door.

"Room seven," she said.

He went to the locker room, changed his clothes, got into his OR togs, and put his hat, smock, and conductive shoes on before entering. The patient was on the operating table. His trach tube was hooked up to the anesthesia machine and a long metal pipe, about three feet long, stuck out of both sides of his upper neck. There was very little bleeding.

"Thanks for coming, Matt," said Dr. Johnson.

"Thanks for inviting me. Has anyone looked down his throat with a laryngoscope?"

"No," said the anesthesiologist. "We felt we needed to get an airway beneath the obstruction."

"Let me borrow your laryngoscope," said Matt. He opened the blade and put it into the patient's throat.

What he saw was a metal pipe that had gone through the neck below the base of the tongue, obstructing any view into the deeper areas of the throat and had come out on the opposite side. There were a few small clots of blood, but he really couldn't see anything.

"Did you put some blood on call? Do we have any blood in the room?"

"We've got one unit in the room," said the anesthesiologist.

"Get another one, just in case. We need to pull the pipe out of his neck, one side at a time. The compression of the pipe has helped to control bleeding. We'll do the right side first. Dr. Perkins, stuff a sterile towel in the center hole of the pipe so as we pull the pipe out the towel will be in the neck. It's like the little Dutch boy with his finger in the dike. The only difference is the sterile towel ends up in the hole. Are we all set to go?" he asked the anesthesiologist.

"I'm as ready as you are," he replied.

"He's had intravenous antibiotics. We have to prep and drape the neck. Someone has to gently pull the pipe from the left side of the neck. Dr. Perkins, you'll do that job. I'll tell you when to start and when to stop."

Everyone assumed their positions. Finally, they were ready to begin.

"Gently pull the pipe, Dr. Perkins. Someone is going to have to steady his head."

The pipe was first greased with sterile bone wax. As the end of the pipe got into the oral cavity, brisk bleeding ensued. Dr. Johnson, the plastic surgeon, and Matt quickly clamped the bleeders and used silk suture ligatures. The hole in the neck was then closed in a layered fashion from the inside out.

The left side of the neck was treated in a similar manner and the pipe was completely removed. The towel was then removed. The bleeding was most brisk on the left side of the neck, so an incision was made and one of the major branches of the carotid artery that goes to the head was pouring out blood. Silk suture ligatures were used to tie the large vessel off and the wound in the left neck was closed.

"Now we'll have a chance to look inside the oral cavity to see what damage has been done," said Matt. "Let me use your laryngoscope again. Also get me my fiberoptic scope so I can get a brighter light into the area."

He put the Jakoscope into the mouth and the lights were put on bright. He put it further down into the throat. There were tears on both sides of the neck. The pipe (about ½ inch in diameter), had been driven through the neck above the vocal chords and cartilages of the neck, anterior to the major blood vessels that went to the head.

"My God, this guy was lucky," said Matt. "He's going to make it. He'll be able to swallow normally and I believe he'll even be able to talk."

"We'd better call his family," the anesthesiologist said.

"Yeah," said Matt. "And while you're at it, call Ripley's."

Matt never caught the gambling bug, but when he moved his golf membership closer to Whitestone Hospital to Whispering Pines Country Club, he noticed there was a poker table in the men's lounge and every Thursday afternoon around 3:30 P.M. a game would begin.

The poker table was reserved for a regular group of players. The members of the group were the president of a large insurance company, the president of a bank, the owner of a small aircraft parts company, the owner of a car dealership, and a respected criminal lawyer.

They played all forms of poker: straight, draw, stud, high-low, high-low seven card stud, and low ball. It was quite confusing at times to the observer, but the players, for all their different backgrounds, played like professionals.

Most of the poker games were dealer's choice. There were certain house rules the five seemed to abide by, and if there was any question about the cards being used, a new deck would be opened. Too much was at stake.

Although each had good days and bad days, the capabilities of the players were essentially even. Some of the players would drop out if they continued to lose, but there was always someone ready to take their place.

After a while, Matt, a neophyte in the world of poker, got to know what hands would win over others: two pair, three of a kind, straight, flush, full house, four of a kind, straight flush, royal flush. He occasionally saw four of a kind but never a straight flush.

One Thursday afternoon, the play was getting rather tense because the president of the insurance company, John Dialer, was raking in all the chips and the rest were doing poorly, and upping the ante trying to recoup their losses. There was no limit to the betting.

Matt was sitting behind the lawyer, Walter Mack, who was not doing well. They were playing straight draw poker, he was the dealer, and would be the last one to bet. The hand was dealt and all five players stayed in as the betting went around. Walt drew an ace, king, queen, and ten of spades, and three of diamonds. There were possibilities there. He discarded the three of diamonds and took one card, and kept it face down on the table in front of him. Two players dropped out. Another player had asked for only one card. The betting went around and the chips piled up. It finally came down to John Dialer and Walter Mack.

It looked like they had both drawn to a straight flush or a full house. Walt peeked at the card on the table and raised the bet by 20 chips. No one was backing off. Either Dialer was bluffing or he had drawn a flush. He raised 20 more and called the bet, now worth about $1,200.

Dialer put his cards face up first. He had a full house; three aces, the ace of hearts, the ace of diamonds, the ace of clubs, and two kings; the king of hearts and the king of diamonds.

Walter Mack had a smile on his face. He had a straight flush; ace, king, queen, jack, and ten of spades—a royal flush! He started to rake in the pot. Suddenly he got pale, looked at Matt and said, "Doc, I feel sick to my stomach. I think I'm going to pass out."

Matt thought he was kidding. He took a closer look at him. There was sweat pouring off his brow and he was ashen. He gripped the edges of the table.

Matt took his pulse and it was rapid. "Have you ever had heart trouble?"

"Heart attack. Five years ago," Walter blurted out.

"We're going to the hospital." He told one of the other poker players to call the emergency room and tell them they were coming in and to have a cardiologist waiting.

"Do we have any O_2 at this country club?"

"No, Doc," said the club attendant.

"Great. One of you guys come with me."

They put Walter into Matt's car. He put his flashers on and kept his hand on the horn as he drove through the red lights on the way to the hospital.

"I want to stop at home. See my wife," said the attorney. "Stop at my house."

"We don't have time for that," said Matt. He was afraid the attorney was going into cardiogenic shock, from a disturbance of his heart rate and rhythm. It is most commonly due to an acute myocardial infarction but can be attributed to other causes. "Try to take normal deep breaths," Matt shouted. The lawyer looked like he was about to pass out.

What Matt was afraid of was that his heart was going into fibrillation and wasn't pumping enough blood to his vital tissues. There would be no oxygen delivery, particularly to the brain, and if shock persisted, the organs in the body would become impaired and there would be irreversible brain damage, then death. The lawyer hung on, and was still conscious when Matt pulled his car up to the ER.

Dr. Donahue, the cardiologist, was there with a stretcher. He was put into the first available room. The crash cart was there, waiting.

Donahue took his blood pressure. His pulse was weak and he was slipping. "We're going to have to zap him," said Donahue.

He placed the positive and negative paddles on his chest and threw the current. Walt's body shook violently and almost flew off the stretcher. His pressure started to come back.

"Somebody get an IV started," hollered Donahue.

"He doesn't have any big veins," said Matt.

"Call anesthesia to pass an endrotracheal tube. He needs oxygen to his lungs and brain."

"Try hitting his femoral vessels in the leg or jugulars," said one of the residents.

"Draw up a bolus of Xylocaine," hollered Donahue.

"We may need a cutdown," hollered Matt.

"Get me a setup, nurse."

One of the residents was able to hit the major vessel in the leg and they injected the bolus of Xylocaine.

"What's his pressure doing now?" asked Donahue.

"It's coming back," said the resident. "He's at 120 systolic. He was down to 50, or zero, maybe."

"He's got a regular heartbeat. Great. Give him some Streptokinase. What's the EKG reading?"

"Elevated S-T segments, but a regular rate now. His pressure's at 160 systolic. He's fighting the endotracheal tube."

Slowly, the lawyer's perimeters returned to normal with IV heart medication and continuous oxygenation.

"We'll put him in the cardiac intensive care unit," said Donahue. "He's had an acute myocardial infarction. If he stabilizes, we'll do an angiogram of his coronary vessels to see where the block is. We'll scan his heart later to see if he's got any good muscle left."

Donahue spoke to Matt. "Two minutes longer and he would have been dead."

Three weeks later an angiogram of the coronary vessels was done. There were multiple areas of blockage. His vessels looked like a moth-eaten rat's tail. A few days later he had a successful five-vessel coronary bypass operation.

A top touring pro, a good friend of the patient, sent him a small palm tree with a bird's nest under it with a golf ball in it. That was an added motivation for the patient to get better.

When Walt got well, he asked Matt what had happened.

"Beats me," said Matt. "But I never knew poker could be life-threatening. You scared the crap out of us all."

"Yeah, I think my riverboat gambler days are done."

"I'd agree with that."

"What happened to the money that I won?"

"We gave it to the bartender and had an open bar for all the members. We figured you were going to die. We thought that would be the way you'd want to be remembered."

"You bastards," he said. "I knew it would be something like that. Well, that was the first royal flush I ever drew in cards and I hope I never draw another one. It almost killed me."

20

"DR. GEORGE HAROLD from St. Mary's Hospital is on the phone," said Judy.

Matt picked up.

"Hello, George. What's going on across town?"

"I'm fighting the cancer battle just like you are," said George. "I've got something to ask you. How would you like to come over to my hospital and help me on a difficult case?"

"It's OK with me, but I don't have operating privileges at your hospital."

"Well, you'll have to get the new Mother Superior's blessing," said George. "I'll talk to her and arrange an interview for you. When can you see her?"

"Set it up for some afternoon and I'll work it out."

Later that afternoon Matt's office got a call and a meeting was set up for him to be interviewed the next week by Sister Mary Margaret, the Mother Superior of St. Mary's Hospital.

On Wednesday afternoon, he drove to St. Mary's Hospital and met Sister Mary Margaret. He had filled out a long application form in her outer office.

"Dr. George Harold thinks you would make an excellent addition to our staff," she said. "What type of surgery do you plan to do?"

"My primary interest is in cancer surgery," said Matt. "Just like his."

"Good. I'm glad to hear that, because I talked to Dr. Simmons, our chief of surgery, and he doesn't want any more general surgeons. He doesn't want you doing the bread and butter cases of the general surgeons—the hernias and gallbladders."

"If I'm busy enough doing tumor surgery, I won't have the occasion

197

to perform that type of surgery. I'm not interested in trauma cases either."

"That's good," said Sister Mary Margaret. "What's your religious preference?"

Matt thought about that. Why was she asking? And what did she want to hear? He believed in God, but in most ways he was liberal when it came to religion. He decided to use Nancy's religion.

"I'm an Episcopalian," said Dr. Kendall. "My wife's father was a bishop."

"That's good," said the Mother Superior. "That's not too far removed from being a Catholic. I'm sure we can expedite your operating room privileges."

With that statement, he was excused.

Two days later, he got a call from Dr. Harold. "They've approved your operating privileges. I want you to help me on a case a week from Monday."

"Let me look at my schedule," said Matt, flipping through his datebook. "What type of case is it?"

"It's a commando procedure on one of our local insurance executives."

"Why do you need me for that one?"

"I want to do a mandible replacement like the one you wrote about in that scientific journal. I read about it and I think I have an ideal patient to use it on."

The day came. The young resident doctors had heard about the procedure. They wanted to watch the new procedure.

The operation went well, with Matt assisting Dr. Harold. When it came time to replace the area in the jaw that had been removed, Matt made an incision over the left pelvic bone and, using a bone cutting saw, cut out a piece of bone the size of the resected jaw. He then took a bone drill and made multiple holes in the outer surface of the bone. He placed the new segment of bone in the resected jaw and, using special wires, anchored the new bone in place. He then used a dental device to fix the jaw in place, so there would be no movement of the fragment of bone in the jaw. Antibiotics were given to prevent infection.

The patient did very well, the jawbone healed, and the dental device was removed six weeks later. The patient had a new lease on life, a symmetrical face. The cosmetic result was excellent.

The word soon got out that it was no longer necessary to send difficult head and neck cancer cases out of state.

Many of the medical directors of major corporations consulted with Matt and, as a result, he took care of many of the C.E.O.s of the major insurance companies and a nearby aircraft engine corporation. He also did a major head and neck operation on the Chairman of the Board of Whitestone Hospital.

His surgical tumor practice flourished.

Three years after doing that case, Matt's relationship with Dr. Harold received a big jolt.

"Matt, this is George. I have a big favor to ask of you."

"What is it?" he asked.

"I've decided to relocate. I'm moving south. I'm going to practice in Florida. I want you to take care of a few of my difficult cancer cases. We don't have any trained surgical oncologists at St. Mary's."

"I'll be glad to. What made you decide to leave?"

"I'm fed up with the new chief of surgery. Life is too short to go through each day with some kind of bullshit harassment. He's from New York City and his ass is tighter than a snare drum. On top of that, he doesn't know how to operate."

"Most of those guys who become chiefs of surgery are politicians and administrators anyway. They know how to operate in the beginning, but they lose their skills when they shuffle paper due to administrative workload. He shouldn't bother you if you're doing your job right."

"Well, he has. He came into my operating room more than once and asked me why I was doing a certain operation. I can't live with that. It's embarrassing. The guy doesn't know how to do the operation himself and he's busting my chops. Forget it. Who needs it?"

"Have you had a frank talk with him, eyeball to eyeball?"

"Yes," said Dr. Harold. "He's an arrogant son of a bitch. He doesn't listen. He's like a freight train going down the railroad tracks. He's on an ego trip. He's like a dictator."

"Well, if he doesn't listen and he's as big a pain in the ass as you say, then you should leave. When are you going?"

"In about six weeks. My wife is in Florida looking for a house right now."

"Well, I'm sorry to see you leave. We've had a good relationship and you've been a good friend. The community is going to miss you. I'll be glad to follow any of your patients."

"Thanks. I'll have my secretary send you a list of patients."

* * *

One of Dr. Harold's patients was a 47-year-old woman, Mrs. Harnet, who was being followed by him for multiple skin cancers of the face. When she was young she saw a dermatologist who gave her radiation treatments for severe acne and she showed evidence of radiation changes over the cheekbones, nose, chin, and lip areas. Dr. Harold had removed several basal cell skin cancers, leaving numerous scars from his surgery.

Matt tried to refer her to a young dermatologist in the area but she refused to go because she felt that a dermatologist had caused her problem in the first place and hadn't kept records of the amount of radiation he had used. Because he didn't keep records she couldn't sue him. Matt was stuck with her.

She had a lot of justifiable bitterness, but because of all the signs she had, one could predict she would have more problems in the future.

That wasn't her only problem. There was a family history of breast cancer. Her mother and twin sister had both died from it. She had multiple lumps in both breasts beginning at age 14. Because of the high risk of breast cancer, Dr. Harold had planned to remove all her breast tissue on both sides and to replace the breast tissue with silicone implants. When the patient was 38 years old, Dr. Harold attempted this, but because of a leaking implant and a severe post-operative infection, the silicone implant had to be removed. The infection persisted for 12 weeks and multiple antibiotics were used to fight it. The infection eventually subsided, leaving her chest flat and scarred. The left breast was not treated because of what had happened to the right.

Her body had been attacked in two areas—her face and right breast, and she was still at a great risk to get cancer of her remaining left breast, given her personal and family history.

Matt was sure there was still breast tissue present in the right chest wall where the implant had to be removed. It was a mess because of what had happened. He wouldn't be able to do a mammogram on that area. He'd have to feel with his fingers for lumps and bumps that could be cancer.

He continued to follow her closely at three-month intervals and, sure enough, a few years later she developed a breast cancer in the left breast which was picked up by a mammogram, and had to have a modified mastectomy. A test used to determine whether her breast cancer bound estrogen and progesterone was done and it was negative. This meant that if she got a recurrent cancer, it would not respond to hormone therapy such as Tamoxifen. This suggested a poor prognosis.

Each year that Matt practiced surgery, he received an increase cost in his malpractice insurance. It blew his mind! All the doctors were at great risk to be sued by a lawyer if an accident occurred. Certain specialties were at greater risk than others: neurosurgery, orthopedics, obstetrics, and general surgery. Their rates were the highest.

Because he was considered an expert in cancer surgery, Matt was often asked by the insurance companies to be an expert witness on pending cancer cases.

Before he would agree to be an expert witness, he would review the legal material to be sure it was not a frivolous lawsuit and the case had merit and had not received damaging attention in the local newspapers. If it was obvious that malpractice or an avoidable accident had taken place, he would advise the principals to settle. It would be a waste of time and money to pursue obvious malpractice.

An expert witness is a no-win proposition. If the doctor being sued loses his case, he would forever blame the witness for the damage done. If he lent his expertise to the defense of a patient, the powers that be in the insurance company would be unhappy.

The real winners in such cases are the lawyers, who collect one-third to 50 percent of the settlement.

In one case, he gave an expert opinion against a law firm specializing in malpractice. Matt brought the trial to an abrupt end with his testimony. The Superior Court Judge asked him whether there was any justification for the malpractice case.

"Your Honor, in all candor, this is a waste of my time and everyone else's in this courtroom. The deceased died on the table from complications unforeseeable by any surgeon."

The judge then told the two opposing lawyers they had one hour to settle the case or he would declare a mistrial and have the case reviewed by the State Legal Ethics Committee. As the lawyers sheepishly adjourned to the hallway, Dr. Kendall could hear pieces of the conversation.

"One-hundred-thousand dollars," said one.

"Ten-thousand dollars," said the other.

"Fifty-thousand dollars."

Time was running out. The judge started to walk over to the lawyers.

"I'll settle for thirty-thousand." The two lawyers shook hands. Each would be compensated for their legal work. Little would be left for the plaintiff.

As Matt walked out of the courtroom, the widow of the deceased stopped him in the hallway. "Your testimony deprived my children of their education."

Matt looked at the woman, a mixture of pity and contempt filling him. "I told the truth. There was no malpractice committed in your husband's case." He walked briskly past her.

Most malpractice cases are settled out of court. In rare instances, a jury decides the outcome. Depositions of expert witnesses and letters between plaintiff and defense are often all that's needed. There was a premium placed on legal bluster and posturing.

Matt was approached by a downstate law firm that specialized in malpractice to review a case and give an expert opinion. The case was a 58-year-old man who had been in an automobile accident. He had a previously known carcinoma of the prostate, and a prominent medical oncologist had testified the auto accident dislodged tumor cells from the quiescent carcinoma, resulting in a diffuse spread of the cancer to the bones of the pelvis and back.

X-rays showed numerous lytic (washed out) areas in his pelvic bones. Blood tests confirmed, in all probability, the bone areas were cancerous. A biopsy of the bone defect was done and it showed prostatic carcinoma. The patient eventually had both testicles removed and was given chemotherapy. He died approximately three years after the accident. His widow, representing her deceased husband's estate, was suing for three million dollars, with the testimony of a prominent medical oncologist to back her.

When the patient had the accident, numerous x-rays were taken in the hospital emergency room. X-rays of the bones of the pelvis and back were taken to check for fractures. However, there was controversy about the findings.

Finally, a date and time for Dr. Kendall's deposition was set.

He was sworn in before a notary public and a court recorder.

"Do you solemnly swear to tell the truth, the whole truth, and nothing but the truth?"

"I do."

"Dr. Kendall, have you ever seen x-rays of bones that show cancer like the case being presented?" asked Attorney White.

"Yes," replied Dr. Kendall.

"Have you seen the x-rays of the bones taken when Mr. Charles was in the emergency room?"

"Yes."

"What do those x-rays show?'

"In my opinion, the x-rays show lytic areas in the large bones of the pelvis."

"What do you mean by lytic areas in the bones?"

"It means there has been a lysis in the area of bone, a washing out of normal bone," replied Matt.

"Are you sure?" asked Attorney White. "A prominent radiologist says he is not sure because there are bowel contents obstructing the views."

"I disagree," said Matt. "Three days later when they repeated the x-rays, there was certainly definite evidence of bone destruction."

"That's exactly what we're talking about," said Attorney White. "Dr. Roberts, the medical oncologist for the plaintiff, says the auto accident spread the cells to cause those x-ray findings."

"I don't believe that! The lytic areas in the bones of the pelvis seen three days after the accident are in the exact area shown on x-rays taken the day of the accident. There needs to be considerable bone destruction, approximately fifty percent, before one can see changes in the bones on plain x-ray films and it takes the body a long time to degenerate to this level before it can be seen on an x-ray."

"How long does it take?" asked Attorney White.

"Several months."

"Are you absolutely sure?" asked Attorney White.

"Absolutely," replied Matt. "Research has been done in trying to get tumors to spread, actually injecting cells with cancer. They were unable to get a take or metastasis that quick. It just doesn't work! If it were true that trauma causes the spread of cancer, then anyone in an auto accident would have to be scrutinized closely. We would see the link."

That case was settled out of court and the plaintiff was sued for instituting a frivolous lawsuit. The plaintiff's expert witness was also sued for false and misleading testimony.

Six months later, Dr. Kendall was asked to review another malpractice case.

Gale Soares was a 30-year-old nurse who was unable to get pregnant. Married for six years, she worked in a small general hospital. When she finally did get pregnant, she went to see a group of obstetricians at her hospital. She was about five months pregnant at the time of her first visit.

Dr. Jones, an obstetrician, checked her and found that she was in good health and the baby was progressing nicely. There was only one small area of concern—she had a one-centimeter, firm, nontender, movable mass in her left breast.

"Gale, we'll have to keep an eye out for any change in that area," he said. "Remind me to check your breasts when you return in four weeks."

"Is there anything to worry about?"

"Not really," said Dr. Jones. "Your breasts have gotten quite a bit larger in preparation for the birth of your child."

Six weeks later, Gale returned for her examination by the group of obstetricians and Dr. Jones was on vacation. Dr. Williams saw her.

"How are things going?"

"Fine, except I feel as big as a truck."

"You've gained quite a bit of weight. You should watch your diet."

Dr. Williams examined her breasts, which had increased in size, and then listened for the fetal heart beat.

"I think everything is okay," he replied.

"I still have that thickness in my left breast," said Gale. She pointed to the area.

Dr. Williams felt the area. "It's hard to tell what's happening in your breasts when they're this large. Do you have a surgeon you might want to see?"

"Dr. Hayes is a friend of the family," said Gale. "I'd feel most comfortable with him."

"I'll give him a call," said Dr. Williams, and picked up the phone. A short conversation ensued, and when he hung up, he said, "Dr. Hayes will see you next Tuesday. Have him send me a report."

Gale went to see Dr. Hayes and after he examined her breasts he said, "It looks like you have a clogged milk duct here. Put some warm moist towels on your breast for twenty minutes, twice a day."

"My aunt had both of her breasts removed for cancer," Gale volunteered.

"Well, this is nothing like that," he said. "When is your due date?"

"In about ten weeks."

"Why don't you come back in three or four weeks and I'll check you again."

"Should I be concerned?"

"No, not at all," replied Dr. Hayes.

Four weeks elapsed and Gale returned.

"You do have some thickening in that left breast," said Dr. Hayes.

"I know that," she said tersely. "I have a neighbor who recently had a breast tumor removed. She told me sometimes they can do a needle biopsy. Should I have one?"

"I don't think it's necessary. We can check you out after you have your baby."

Four weeks later, Gale went into labor. The delivery was rough, and a caesarean section was performed. She delivered a 7½ pound healthy baby boy and asked Dr. Jones if she could breastfeed her baby.

"I don't see why not," he replied.

So she did, for five weeks. She noted the lump in her left breast increased in size. She decided to call Dr. Jones.

"I think you better see Dr. Hayes," he said.

She made an appointment with Dr. Hayes and when she saw him his comment was, "You've got a good-sized mass in this breast. Where have you been?"

"Where have I been? This is the third time I've seen you."

"Oh, that's right. That lump is the size of a hen's egg. You need to have it removed to see what it is."

"I guess I'll have to stop nursing."

"That's right."

Arrangements were made, she was taken to the operating room the following week, and the large mass was removed. It was diagnosed as an infiltrating ductal carcinoma. Because of the size of the tumor, she was advised to have her breast removed along with a sampling of the axillary glands, known as a modified mastectomy and axillary dissection.

She agreed to the operation. The breast was removed and the glands were sampled to see if the cancer had spread. Examination of the tissue revealed seven glands involved with cancer. Shattered, she returned to the doctor who had escorted her into this disaster.

"Am I going to die?" she asked Dr. Hayes.

"We're going to do everything we can to keep you alive," he said. "You're going to need chemotherapy and possibly radiation."

"Will I lose my hair?"

"Only for a short while," he replied.

"I'm not so sure I want chemotherapy. I think I'm going to get a second opinion."

"That's fine with me. I'll get your records ready for you to take with you."

She and her husband went to New York City to a major cancer center where she was advised to have chemotherapy.

Two years after her surgery and chemotherapy, she developed diffuse metastases to the spine, ribs and skull, and died six months later.

Prior to her death, a video was made. In it, she described her relationship with the group of obstetricians and the surgeon. She stated she had told the obstetricians that her mother and aunt both had breast cancer. She also told them she had three uncles who had died of cancer. She stated she had asked Dr. Hayes on two occasions about whether she needed a mammogram, and also suggested that a neighbor had told her to mention needle biopsy. None of these facts were heeded.

Ricardo, Stevens and Dunbar, one of the leading law firms in the state, asked Matt if he would consider taking the case.

He said he'd review the chart.

After his review, he agreed to help the plaintiff. The same day a lawyer for the insurance company called him and asked if he would defend the doctors.

"Sorry," said Matt, "I'm on the other side of this one. The standard of medical care was shoddy, and breast cancer is a field I have some expertise in."

"We'll see you in court," said the lawyer.

Two weeks later, Matt was notified that a deposition concerning the case would take place in the legal offices of the defendant's lawyer. Both law firms would be represented and the deposition would be under oath.

Matt was sworn in by a notary public.

Q. "Dr. Kendall, what is your present position at your hospital?"
A. "I am a senior surgical oncologist on the staff at Whitestone Hospital."
Q. "Are you in private practice?"
A. "Yes."
Q. "What qualifies you to be an expert witness in this case?"
A. "My education and professional experience."

Attorney Atwood, sitting next to Dr. Kendall, spoke up. "Objection. I have given you Dr. Kendall's curriculum vitae. It shows he has written many articles on cancer in the medical literature and has been the past president of local, state, and regional cancer societies. He's also written a book about breast cancer. He is amply qualified."

"I agree," said Attorney Scully. "However, I want his qualifications on the record. If you will accept using the written documents as part of the deposition, I'll change the questioning."

"Fine," said Atwood.

Q. "Dr. Kendall, is it difficult to detect breast cancer in a woman who is pregnant?"
A. "It can be, depending on what trimester of the pregnancy she is in. It's easier to detect cancer in the first three months than in the last three months."
Q. "Does obesity play a role in the detection of breast cancer?"
A. "Until recently it did. You had to feel it and detect it by direct examination and obviously it's more difficult to detect a breast tumor in an obese patient."
Q. "Was the patient we are discussing obese?"
A. "From reading the records I would say so. She weighed over 200 pounds."
Q. "So it would be difficult for the doctor to feel any changes?"
A. "That's right. But, the patient said she felt changes and more than one medical observer agreed with her."
Q. "If your wife was obese, pregnant, and told you she had a breast lump, what would you do?"
A. "I'd treat her like she wasn't pregnant, with a few reservations. I'd do a mammogram, and if there was a lump, I'd do a needle biopsy or open biopsy of it. I'd also tell the radiologist to protect the abdomen with a lead shield so the unborn baby would not be exposed to radiation."

Q. "What if she had a cancer? How would you treat her?"
A. "It would depend on when it was discovered. Also, with some patients, it might depend on their religious preference.
Q. "Would you clarify that?"
A. "If the lump was found early and it was small, she could have a lumpectomy and axillary dissection. If the lump was found later, say at eight months, and if the baby was big enough, a caesarean section might be recommended. In some cases, if the tumor was found in the first three months, some doctors might even recommend the pregnancy be terminated."
Q. "What about you?"
A. "If the cancer developed within the first three months, I might consider recommending an abortion but probably not if she was any further into the pregnancy."
Q. "Why not?"
A. "It's my own personal feeling."
Q. "Do you feel malpractice has occurred in this case?"
A. "That's for the lawyers and judge to decide."
Q. "That's not true. Let me put it another way. Was the case of this patient up to the standard of care given in this community by other physicians?"
A. "I would have to say no. There was a critical delay in diagnosis and treatment. Both the obstetricians and surgeons were at fault. The continuity of care was poor. There should have been a higher degree of attention and diligence because she was in a high-risk group with her family history of breast cancer."

A month later, Matt gave the same testimony in the courtroom in front of a jury. Once the jury heard Matt's testimony, it was obvious that the defense was in big trouble. The doctors had not taken care of the pregnant woman properly when she got her breast cancer. There was obvious delay in diagnosis that contributed to her early demise. The case was settled for a large sum.

21

On a midsummer Sunday afternoon, while Matt was relaxing at home with Nancy, he received a call from an emergency walk-in clinic 60 miles away. A nurse was on the phone.

"Dr. Kendall, we have a breast cancer patient of yours here in our clinic, a Mrs. Harnet."

"What's wrong with her?"

"She fractured her left arm trying to open a window at her cottage. Her relative, Dr. Pesto, an orthopedic surgeon, brought her here."

"Let me talk to him."

"Dr. Kendall, this is Dr. Pesto. Mrs. Harnet fractured her left arm trying to open a stuck window."

"What does the x-ray show?"

"It shows a hairline fracture of her left humerus," he replied.

"She'll have to be worked up for metastatic bone disease. Take her to the emergency room at Whitestone Hospital. We'll have her admitted."

"She's comfortable. I gave her some pain medication and put her arm in a tight Velpeau sling. She doesn't want to go into the hospital. You can see her tomorrow."

"I'm not a bone specialist. Do you want to take care of her?"

"No. Have one of your orthopedic men at Whitestone see her. Dr. Sloan, the chief of orthopedics, would be good."

"I'll see if he's available. Tell Mrs. Harnet that I'll see her at 2:00 P.M. tomorrow in my office."

Matt examined Mrs. Harnet when she came into his office on Monday afternoon. Her arm was in a tight sling, she appeared quite pale, and obviously had quite a bit of pain in her upper arm. Judy was with him when he examined her.

209

"Tell me what happened," he said.

"I tried to open the kitchen window at our cottage and it wouldn't budge. I was so mad I banged on the window with my arm as hard as I could and I felt something give. Not in the window, in my arm. My arm hurt like the dickens. I called my daughter and we called a relative, Dr. Pesto, who is a bone specialist. He lives in a cottage nearby. He took me to a clinic and I had x-rays taken. They found out I had a fractured arm."

"I'll admit you to the hospital right away. I discussed having a doctor see you with Dr. Pesto and he suggested Dr. Sloan, the chief of orthopedics."

"I don't want to go into the hospital today. I hate hospitals."

"You need to have some studies done."

"I'm sorry, I can't go today."

"You have to go in tomorrow morning, then. We have to find out why you broke your arm."

"If I have to go in, I'll go, but I don't like it."

The next morning, Mrs. Harnet was admitted. The surgical resident took a history, did a physical, and documented her problems. She told him about the multiple recurrent basal cell cancers of the face she had and her long course of breast problems starting when she was a teenager. She had numerous lumps in both breasts with fibrocystic disease for many years. She told him that when she was 40, both breasts were to be removed to prevent breast cancer.

The operation was to be done in two stages, she stated, with the right breast being done first. Unfortunately, the silicone implant that was put in leaked. "I got an overwhelming infection and they had to take the silicone implant out. I was in the hospital for eight weeks.

"I've had to live with a horrible flat chest on that side all my life. That was a great operation by my surgeon at St. Mary's. I hate him! I should have sued him. My husband, who's a lawyer, said I should have, too! The only reason I didn't was because he was a friend of the family and went to our church. I developed cancer in my left breast four and a half years ago, which was treated by Dr. Kendall. He took that one off. Now I'm flat-chested. I don't think any man would be interested in having sex with me."

The surgical intern continued to take the history and record it in the chart. The scenario got more interesting.

"My mother died of ovarian cancer and my twin sister died three years ago of breast cancer. I also had two aunts who had breast cancer."

Incredible, thought the resident. This woman's a walking time bomb.

After taking the history, Dr. Scott had her disrobe and he began the physical examination.

What a mess! Her face had scars from repeated surgery for skin cancer. She had radiation damage to both sides of her face, with little spider-like blood vessels all over her cheeks. She was chronically depressed. One look could tell you that.

Her right chest wall, where she had the attempted surgery to remove the breast tissue, followed by the infection and removal of the silicone implant, had a flat, distorted appearance. There was also a large scar from the left mastectomy.

"It's not a pretty sight for a young doctor to see, is it?"

Dr. Scott, the young resident, was afraid to answer that question honestly. He hesitated for quite a while and finally blurted out. "I've seen worse."

He listened to her heart, took her blood pressure, and examined her abdomen. It wasn't easy to do because of her fractured arm. He finally completed the physical exam.

At the bottom of the chart was a space for filling in a working diagnosis. He didn't know whether to put her psychological problems down first or her cancer problems. He finally wrote;

1. Fracture of the right arm, question of metastatic breast cancer.
2. Multiple basal cell cancers of the face, secondary to damage from radiation treatments for acne.
3. Chronic depression, secondary to above.

When Dr. Scott got out to the nurses' station he filled out a consultation form for Dr. Sloan. He called Sloan's office. The secretary said he would see her that afternoon.

Sloan was a middle-aged Phi Beta Kappa from Yale, with a medical degree from Harvard. He had taken his residency in bone surgery at Mass General. He had a tendency to be arrogant, very gruff, and rigid. Usually he had an entourage of young doctors in training around him, who did not speak unless spoken to.

"Well, young lady, I hear you tried to break a window at your cottage. Instead you broke your arm. How's the pain?"

"Awful."

"That can be controlled with shots and pills."

"How often can I have them?" she asked.

"What's she getting?" Dr. Sloan asked the head nurse.

"Seventy-five milligrams of Demerol every three hours," she replied.

"Hm, quite a bit. Why so much?"

"She's had multiple medications in the past for other problems."

"Well, keep her comfortable. Have the pain people see her. Mrs. Harnet, we're going to do some studies to make sure the break in your arm isn't due to cancer." There was a broad smile on his face.

"That's great," said Mrs. Harnet. "But why are you smiling?"

"I'm not smiling," replied Dr. Sloan, as his expression changed.

It looked like a smile to Mrs. Harnet. What a great bedside manner, she thought.

Sloan shrugged and plowed on with what he knew best—medicine.

"What you've got is a clean break in the bone in your upper arm, the spot showing up where the fracture is, is really nothing. Dr. Kendall and I are going to do some tests to be sure the break in your arm is due to trauma and not cancer. Has Dr. Kendall been in to see you?"

"Yes," said Mrs. Harnet. "He said he was going to do a bone scan and liver scan in the next two days to make sure the breast tumor hadn't spread."

"Fine," said Dr. Sloan. "I've reviewed your x-ray films with some of my colleagues. Those bones are in good alignment. It's a thin hairline fracture so we won't have to do anything except have you wear the restraining sling and restrict your activities. We'll be sure to keep you comfortable with pain medication. These young resident doctors will be keeping an eye on you also."

During the next two days, a bone scan to check all the bones in her body was done. A radioactive dye was injected into her veins and the dye concentrated in her bones. A Geiger-counter type instrument was then used to outline her bone structures. The study showed only one hot spot, at the site of the fracture. This was expected. The rest of her bones were normal. A similar study was done on her liver and showed no evidence of disease.

Dr. Sloan and his entourage saw her the morning of her discharge.

"Everything turned out all right for you, young lady. However, I don't want you banging on any cottage windows anymore. It'll take you three or four months to completely heal that bone. I'll see you in my office in a week and we'll schedule follow-up visits. Dr. Kendall wants to see you periodically also to make sure you don't get into trouble. Give his office a call."

Matt also saw Mrs. Harnet before discharge. He worried about her. She was not good about coming in for follow-up visits.

"I've talked to Dr. Sloan about you. He told me he felt that you have a traumatic fracture and that the bone scan and liver scan are negative for cancer. That's good! I want you to come and see me in my office after you heal that arm. You'll have to be watched closely."

"Why do I have to see you? I'm going to be seeing Dr. Sloan."

"That's up to you. You still should be followed for your breast cancer."

Mrs. Harnet came in three months after her bone had been broken. She was doing well and was more concerned with her facial skin cancers than her arm.

Three months later, she was seen again with few complaints, but a follow-up card had to be sent to get her to return to the office.

After another three months, Judy had to send another follow-up card to Mrs. Harnet because she didn't show up. There was no response.

Dr. Kendall completed his last operative case Friday and looked up at the clock. It was 1:00 P.M. Joyce, his circulating nurse, untied his waterproof surgical gown in the back. He removed it, and threw it into a special laundry container.

When he got to his office, he had lunch with Judy and briefly discussed the operative cases and pertinent phone calls.

"You have a surprise in store for you this afternoon."

"What do you mean?"

"Wait and see. You have a PITA coming in today."

"I don't like those cases you call PITAs," said Matt.

"They're what you call *pains in the ass*, to put it more plainly," replied Judy. "It's Mrs. Harnet."

"I can't disagree with you on that one. But you know we do have a lot of very nice patients."

"That's right. And it's a good thing the nice ones outnumber the others."

After finishing his sandwich, Dr. Kendall started his afternoon office hours.

Near the door of each examining room was a plastic chart holder. He would pick up the chart and glance through it before entering.

After seeing six patients he picked up a thick chart, on Mrs. Harnet.

He opened the door and said, "Good to see you, Helen," as he held out his hand. "It's a nice day."

She didn't return the gesture. "What's so nice about it?" She replied.

"It looks like the weather's nice outside."

"It's cold as hell outside, Doctor. It's January, just in case you haven't noticed. If it weren't for all these skin cancers on my face, I'd be down in Florida trying to get a tan."

"That's right. You do have to watch out for the sun. I want you to lie back on the examining table so I can examine you."

Dr. Kendall felt her chest wall for possible nodules and her armpits and above her clavicles for glands. There were none to be felt. He felt under her right rib cage for her liver. There didn't seem to be any enlargement.

"How do you feel?"

"The same as I've always felt—lousy and depressed."

"Have you seen Dr. Sloan?"

"I saw him in October. He took some x-rays and told me the arm was better and to come back if I broke another bone."

Matt noted on her chart that it had been 14 weeks since he had seen her last. She had been due seven weeks earlier.

"You should come in for follow-up when you're supposed to," he said.

"You're not my favorite doctor. I get nervous before I come in here—every time! I also get pains in the pit of my stomach and I worry about what you may find. Are you through?"

"Yes."

When Dr. Kendall got out of the examining room, Karen, the nurse who had been in there with them, remarked, "That one's worse than a pain in the ass. She's really got a chip on her shoulder."

"You have to feel sorry for her. Make sure Judy gives her a follow-up appointment."

22

THE ORTHOPEDIC DEPARTMENT at Whitestone Hospital consisted of a large group practice of 15 specialists. The chief of orthopedics, Dr. Richard Sloan, had two secretaries—one for handling the administrative duties of the department and the other to handle his medical practice.

Angela Granata, Dr. Sloan's medical secretary and office manager, had worked for him for 20 years and was a tough cookie. She knew how to answer the phone and how to handle difficult problems.

On a day when the phone had been ringing constantly, Angie picked it up and a voice on the other end said, "Why don't you girls stop taking your phones off the hook so a sick patient can make an appointment? I've been trying to get through for fifteen minutes. Where the hell have you been?"

Angie was about to slam the phone back down on the hook but thought better of it. The voice was familiar to her but she wasn't sure who it was. "Who's calling, please?"

"My name is Helen Harnet and I've developed severe pain in my left upper arm. I need an appointment to see the doctor right away!"

When a patient tries to pull a stunt like that to get an early appointment, Angie just makes them wait longer.

"We're very busy now and we're overbooked. The earliest appointment I can give you is in three weeks. Have you seen your family doctor?"

"No. And I don't plan to! Don't give me that bullshit! I've had a fractured arm that Dr. Sloan took care of and it's either broken or something else has gone wrong. I'm in agony, for God's sake! I have to be seen right now!" she screamed.

"Hold for a minute. I have a call on the other line." Angie got out the chart on Mrs. Harnet. She remembered that she had been horrible to take care of.

"We'll try to work you in this afternoon between patients."

When Mrs. Harnet got into Dr. Sloan's office Angie had the nurse put her into an examining room. Dr. Sloan was busy and saw her an hour later.

He looked at her chart and then at Mrs. Harnet and said, "Oh, yes, you're the one who's so afraid of cancer." He then looked at her arm, which was quite painful to touch and appeared swollen.

"We'll need to take some x-rays to see what's going on here," he said. "I hope you haven't banged on any more windows."

"No, I haven't! That's absurd! My arm has been swollen for quite a while."

"Where have you been?" asked Sloan sarcastically.

"Where do you think? Staying away from doctors. That's where! Every time I see you guys I have trouble."

"The x-ray technician will take some x-rays. I'll be back after I look at them."

After the x-rays were developed, Dr. Sloan saw a small lytic area at the site of her previous fracture. He showed the films to a couple of his colleagues. They all agreed that she had a problem.

"I'm sorry I have to tell you this, but it looks as if you have a tumor at the site of your previous fracture. I'll give Dr. Kendall a call."

Sloan went into his consultation room and called Matt. The door to the examining room was inadvertently left open and Mrs. Harnet could hear the whole conversation.

"Matt, you know that Mrs. Harnet you sent me last summer? She's in big trouble! She's got a small moth-eaten area at her old fracture site."

"You'd better order a bone scan and a liver scan," said Matt.

Sloan went back to the examining room and said, "I've talked to Dr. Kendall and he wants you to have liver and bone scans.

"I knew I had a problem," said Mrs. Harnet. "I'm smarter than you guys."

Sloan talked to the head of the nuclear medicine department and the scans were completed within three days. The bone scan showed that there was a small area of change at the fracture site of the left upper arm. The rest of her bones were normal and the liver was unremarkable. Sloan told her to see Dr. Kendall.

When she saw Kendall, she told him what had happened. She included her opinion of Sloan. "That man is an irretrievable asshole. He's the poorest excuse for a doctor I've ever seen. I never want to see him again."

Matt was shocked by Mrs. Harnet's language.

She looked depressed. Dr. Kendall put his arm around her shoulder and said, "It's not the end of the world, Helen. You'll probably need x-ray treatment to that area in your arm. I'll call Bill Andrews, the chief of radiation therapy, and discuss your case with him. Is that all right with you?"

"By all means," she said. "Anything to relieve this pain. However, I don't like the idea of more radiation. Do I have a choice? Look what it did to my face. It seems like that's when all my problems started—with radiation treatments."

Matt called Andrews and told him about Mrs. Harnet's arm.

"I've already seen her x-rays," said Andrews. Sloan asked me to look at them. It looks like a solitary lesion. However, it still could be a primary bone cancer and not a spread from her breast. Those x-ray films aren't clear. It's a tough one to call. I understand she's a heavy smoker. She could have a lung cancer."

"We'd better get a tissue diagnosis then. Get one of your hotshots to do a needle biopsy."

"OK. I'll schedule it."

The next week, the needle biopsy was done. The radiologist had a difficult time getting sufficient tissue for study. He had to stick her three or four times. Mrs. Harnet screamed and kicked and swore at him. She had to be heavily sedated when it was done and had to be hospitalized overnight.

When the tissue was analyzed it showed cancer that was compatible with a breast primary.

Matt went in to see her the day after the biopsy. Mrs. Harnet was quite agitated. "I hate Dr. Sloan. I don't like you either because of the tests you order and that radiologist is from the dark ages. They should have knocked me out before they used those needles."

"I don't blame you for feeling that way. But sometimes you have to do tests that are uncomfortable. I want you to see a good medical oncologist. You'll need chemotherapy and radiation. Think positive. Do you want some names?"

"Dr. Pesto will select someone for me," she replied. "You made a poor choice when you selected Sloan."

"That's fine. But if you'll remember, it was Dr. Pesto who chose Dr. Sloan for you, not me."

"Well, whatever. I still don't like him."

"When you see a medical oncologist have him send me a report." Matt did not hear from him.

Six months later, he received a report from Dr. Dudley, a medical oncologist on the staff of St. Mary's Hospital. He reported that Mrs. Harnet had another bone scan the week before and it now showed diffuse involvement of her skull, back, hips, and ribs with metastatic disease. Her liver was also riddled. He finally started her on chemotherapy.

Two weeks after he received the report from Dr. Dudley, Matt was paged at the hospital. He picked up a phone at the nurses' station and called his hotline number. It was Judy.

"Dr. Kendall, we have a problem here. There's a sheriff with a paper to subpoena Mrs. Harnet's records."

"Well, you'll have to make a copy of the chart and give it to him."

"Her chart's bigger than a dictionary. It'll take me forever to copy it. Don't you want to review the records first?"

"I've got nothing to hide. My only regret is that I had to take care of that lady. I'll review the chart after you make the copies for the sheriff. We'll also have to call our malpractice insurance carrier."

Judy copied the records and gave them to the sheriff.

Later that day, Matt called his insurance carrier and was told that a lawyer would be assigned to the case and would talk to him, once they received the complaint. One month later, he received a copy of the complaint. He and Dr. Sloan, the chief of orthopedics, were the defendants. The plaintiffs were Mrs. Harnet and her husband Philip.

This was the first malpractice suit filed against Dr. Kendall since he had started practice 25 years ago. There were five pages of complaints against him and Dr. Sloan. The suit was for "in excess of one million dollars."

As he read down the sheet of complaints, Matt spiraled downward to anger and sadness. The joy and rewards of practicing medicine were gone.

Mrs. Harnet claimed that after she broke her arm, she had persistent pain and swelling which was a symptom of cancer, and that despite her past history, the defendants failed to exercise due care to diagnose cancer or refer her to a specialist for the proper treatment of her condition.

What did she expect? Matt thought. I am a specialist and I admitted her to the hospital for an extensive work-up. Bone scans and liver scans were negative. I called in the top orthopedic surgeon in the area and he said it was a clean break when she broke her arm. She never came back on time for follow-ups. She never complained about her arm. Her complaints were always about the skin cancers on her face.

Matt continued to read down the list of complaints.

As a result of the plaintiff's injuries, she has been required to expend and will be required to continue to expend considerable sums of money for hospitalization, medication, and medical care and treatment, all to her personal financial loss.

She's made me responsible for the spread of her cancer, thought Matt, and she wants me to pay all her bills out of my malpractice insurance.

As he continued to read down the list, he couldn't believe what she was alleging. The payoff came when he got to the fourth count. Philip Harnet vs. Matt Kendall, M.D.

The plaintiff, Philip Harnet, was at the time of the occurrence and still remains the husband of the plaintiff, Helen Harnet. As a result of the carelessness and negligence of the defendants, Matt Kendall, M.D., and Richard Sloan, M.D., the plaintiff Philip Harnet was deprived of his right to consortium with his wife, the plaintiff, Helen Harnet, including the loss and diminution of companionship, society, affection, sexual relations and moral support afforded by virtue of the marital cohabitation of the plaintiff, Philip Harnet and plaintiff, Helen Harnet, as husband and wife.

"That's great," said Matt. "I suppose I'm responsible for his unhappy sex life, thirty-five years after his marriage."

"It sounds that way," said Judy. "Mrs. Harnet's suing everyone involved with the case. Dr. Bill Henry's office called. He's the radiologist who looked at the x-rays of the fractured arm. He received a subpoena also. He wants you to call him."

"Well, they usually sue everyone involved. It looks like I'm going to be spending a lot of time trying to defend myself in court. I hope they give me a good lawyer."

The hospital Litigation Committee reviewed the case and decided it should be defended because it felt no malpractice had occurred. A prominent law firm was assigned to the case and it wasn't long before

Matt received a call from a lawyer who would be defending him. Her name was Suzanne Bodman, a young, aggressive malpractice lawyer with good credentials.

She had graduated from Harvard Law near the top of her class. She called Matt and arranged to meet with him to discuss the case at his office. Attorney Bodman was an attractive redhead, about 50 years old.

"Dr. Kendall, I've reviewed the records in this case and I must say I'm impressed that you have typed office follow-up records. Most doctors' records are handwritten and you can't read them. Sometimes that's an advantage, if you're a defendant."

"I've got nothing to hide. Now tell me how I can be of help. This is the first time I've ever been sued. Tell me, what's going to happen next?"

"Well, probably an interrogatory or a deposition will be taken from the patient, her husband, daughter, and her relative, the orthopedic surgeon."

"That's great. Why doesn't she sue Dr. Pesto? He was supposed to be following along in her care with the rest of us."

"I'm sure he'll be a hostile witness," said Attorney Bodman. "He could be orchestrating the whole plot. Now, there are a few details I want to ask you about. I also must remind you not to speak to anyone about this case except your legal representative. You're not to discuss the case with Dr. Sloan, either.

"I've reviewed the case and I don't feel any malpractice took place. However, we may have to prove that to a jury. They've taken a videotape of Mrs. Harnet with her pronounced weight loss and gross pictures of her chest. You know what she looks like. I'm sure they plan to show the video to the jury in case she dies.

"In order to prove malpractice, Dr. Kendall, they have to prove that you did not conform to the practice of medicine that takes place in this community. We may need to have some national expert review this case in order to defend you. Do you know anyone who might give an unbiased opinion?"

"I'll have to think about that. I've sat on committees of a few national cancer organizations and know a few bigshots."

"THREE MILLION SUIT FOR MALPRACTICE," was the headline across the front page of the *Whitestone Times*.

"The local law firm of Gottlick, Drucker, Cummings, and Golden announced that their client, Mrs. Helen Harnet, is suing Dr. Matt Kendall, a senior surgeon on the staff of Whitestone Hospital.

"When Mr. Drayton, the hospital's public relations officer, was asked to make a statement about the case, he refused to comment, except to say, 'The hospital is backing its top cancer surgeon, and will support Dr. Kendall in clearing his name of any wrongdoing.' Dr. Kendall is the former president of the State Cancer Society and has served as Chairman of the Cancer Commission for New England.

"Dr. Kendall's office was contacted, but would make no comment on the pending suit.

"The law firm of Chase, Newell, White and Jaworski, which represents Dr. Kendall, has submitted an objection to the Superior Court concerning the announcement of the malpractice case, stating that it would be impossible to get an impartial jury for the trial because of the *Times'* publication of statements by the patient's family. Kendall may ask for a change of venue.

"The *Times'* lawyer, John Brainard, has stated that the paper will continue to publish articles concerning the case, citing the First Amendment. Brainard said all facts concerning the case will be checked prior to publication, sources of information will be protected, and nothing will be published to prejudice the jury. Because of the large amount of money involved in the case, the story, he claimed, is newsworthy.

"Dr. Kendall's office was asked to give a written statement, which the *Times* offered to print in its entirety. Kendall's attorney has advised him not to reply, since any statement might be misinterpreted and the trial could be jeopardized.

"Depositions of the principals in the case will take place soon.

"Expert witnesses from outside the local community, perhaps from New York City or Boston, will be asked to express opinions about the care provided by Kendall in the management of this complex medical case.

"There is some question as to whether Kendall himself will be asked to testify on his own behalf. Dr. Kendall, who has testified as an expert witness in numerous malpractice cases around the country, may not be called by the prosecution for fear of his experience on the stand.

"The trial is scheduled to begin in eight weeks."

When Matt got home from the hospital Nancy was waiting for him at the door when he got out of his car.

"What a horrible day!" said Matt.

"I know, honey," said his wife. Her hands were shaking.

"When I went into medicine, I decided to devote my life to helping the sick. I try to help someone who has cancer, to the best of my ability, I keep her alive for more than five years, and then she turns around and sues me.

"What motivates people to do things like this? I didn't give her her cancer. In fact, I inherited her case from a colleague. I knew she was going to be bad news the first time I saw her.

"In fact, Judy told me not to take the case from that surgeon at St. Mary's when he retired. I should have listened to her."

"Honey, you and I both know you saved her life and kept her alive for a long time."

"I blame part of what's happened on the lawyers," said Matt. "They could give a damn about the patient. They're only interested in money. Sometimes I wish I hadn't stayed in private practice. I should have taken that job as chief of surgery out in the midwest. Then, at least if something happened, the hospital would have to pay. I thought I was Superman. I thought I was too smart and too good to get sued. Wrong! If you're a busy surgeon and you see enough patients, you'll eventually get sued. Doing radical surgery for cancer puts you on the front line and I always liked the way everybody looked up to me like I was God. I felt that sense of power, of doing good. But I'm vulnerable as hell now and I—look at me, I'm shaking."

"That's a normal reaction," said Nancy.

"What bothers me is that everyone at the hospital, including my patients and all of my friends, know I'm being sued. It's a tremendous blow to my ego and my self-confidence has been destroyed. To be a surgeon you have to have confidence, but after this, I don't know. My integrity is going to be permanently damaged, whether I win or lose.

"You don't win all the time, even if you're right. The jury decides what the outcome is. Unfortunately, juries are not made up of doctors, they're laypeople and more often than not, they don't understand. They see the maimed and injured and think you created it."

Nancy nodded assent. "Honey, we'll just have to pray and trust in God that everything will turn out all right."

"I don't know," said Matt. "Your faith is stronger than mine. Why am I getting sued? Is God the one behind the lawsuit?"

"No—it could be the devil, however."

Nancy took his arm and gently pulled him inside the house. They sat together on the sofa in the living room. Out of a long silence, Matt spoke again.

"In order to practice complicated medicine today, so many costly tests are done just so the doctor can protect himself and say, I did that ultrasound test, I did that CT scan—even though they showed nothing. The art of practicing medicine is being mechanized. It's becoming defensive and the cost is skyrocketing.

"Who pays for it?" hollered Matt. "Everyone who pays the practicing doctor and everyone who pays the premium for health insurance. Billions of dollars a year are spent for malpractice insurance and billions of dollars more are spent for the technology to avoid liability. We're the only country that has this problem.

"In England, if you institute a malpractice lawsuit and lose, you pay the cost of the court for both sides. It makes you think twice before you sue someone. The problem is that we have more lawyers in this country then any other country in the world." Finally, he stopped.

"Honey, I'm sorry about what has happened," said Nancy. "I'm sure your reputation has been tarnished, even though the case hasn't gone to trial. You have to keep a stiff upper lip. You've done so much good. Your patients know you have, I know you have, and in your heart, you know you have."

He looked at Nancy, thinking. She's in this, too. Almost as deep as me. "You're the best friend I've got."

23

As the county's legal wheels slowly ground out the procedures for the malpractice case, Matt continued his routine day-to-day surgery. Month after month went by with little progress in the lawsuit.

Attorney Bodman had called Matt and told him she had filed written interrogatories and requests for production to Mrs. Harnet—a way for the defense to ask questions concerning the complaint made against him before going into court. It was a pretrial discovery tool, in which written questions by one party are served on the adversary, who must answer by written replies made under oath. Interrogatories are not as flexible as depositions, which include opportunity for cross examination, but are regarded as a good and inexpensive means of establishing important facts.

Dr. Kendall had suggested to Bodman that he would have liked to ask some specific questions of his patient, Mrs. Harnet, because he couldn't understand why she was blatantly lying. He wanted to talk to her face to face. In fact, he had felt like punching her in the nose.

Attorney Bodman's response was; "We'll have our chance to do that later on when we cross-examine her in a deposition. And punching her in the nose would only cause you intolerable legal trouble in trying to settle this dispute. It would disclose a part of your character that we might not want them to see."

"Well, she's certainly changed my personality, I'll give you that! Many doctors would have discharged her because of her actions. She was a real bitch to take care of. They wouldn't have taken the risk I took. I was sincerely trying to help that lady."

"I know what you're thinking and I appreciate what you're going through. I want you to know that! That's why I took your case. I don't like to lose! We are just beginning to find out what actually happened."

Dr. Kendall kept thinking about the conversation he had with his lawyer as he gently opened the package and took out a thick pile of papers. Judy was standing next to him as he opened it. There was a brief note on top of the papers signed by Attorney Suzanne Bodman.

It read:

Personal and Confidential.

Re: Philip Harnet and Helen Harnet et al vs.
    Matt Kendall, M.D. et al.

Dear Dr. Kendall,

We filed written interrogatories and requests for production upon Mrs. Harnet and have finally received responses. Included in the medical records and other information provided to us were statements made by Mrs. Harnet and other members of her family.

I would be interested in your comments after you have read this material. I have highlighted some of the statements which may need further clarification in a deposition. Please don't hesitate to contact me at any time regarding this matter.

Very truly yours,

Suzanne Bodman
Chase, Newell, White,
Jaworski

SB:jp
Enclosures

STATEMENT BY: Mrs. Harnet

On the August morning in question, around 7:30 A.M., I was in the kitchen of my cottage with my husband. It was raining and it was stuffy inside. I wanted to open the kitchen window because it was muggy and hot, so I got up on a chair to try to push it open. It wouldn't budge so I tried to bang on it to loosen it. I hit it as hard as I could and finally got it opened and got down from the chair. I bent down to pick something up off the floor and I felt an excruciating pain. I heard the bone in my arm snap. I got sick to my stomach and told my husband what had happened. He helped me up and sat me down. My grandson and daughter were also at the cottage and my daughter was directly over the kitchen upstairs and could hear the snap. The pain was so excruciating I couldn't scream or cry. I was breathless.

We called a relative, Dr. Pesto, who is an orthopedic surgeon. He looked at me and called a walk-in clinic nearby so I could have some x-rays taken.

He didn't like the way they looked and was afraid it might be cancer. He called Dr. Kendall and expressed his concern. Dr. Kendall was very surprised and said he didn't know how this could be possible because he had just seen me a few weeks ago for a checkup. He did say, however, that I should be admitted to the hospital immediately.

I was admitted two days later for blood tests, bone scan, liver scan, and x-rays of the left arm. The following day I was told by a resident surgeon that Dr. Kendall had called in Dr. Richard Sloan, the chief of orthopedics, to see me. Dr. Sloan told me that in his opinion there was nothing to be concerned about. The x-rays showed I had a hairline fracture.

I left the hospital the following morning without hearing the results of the bone scan. The liver scan was negative. I eventually found out that the fracture in my arm lit up, which is completely normal for any fracture or injury to bone. There were no other bone abnormalities.

I made an appointment to see Dr. Sloan in late September. When Sloan came into the room on that visit he said to me, "I thought you would be going back to see your relative, Dr. Pesto." I was quite surprised at his statement. I told him the reason I was there was because Dr. Kendall insisted I see him. He took x-rays and said the bone was healing well. I had one more appointment with Dr. Sloan in October when he recommended I go for physical therapy for several weeks, which he extended for another couple of weeks. I remember asking Dr. Sloan when he would like to see me again. He remarked, "Come back and see me if and when you break another bone. You're completely healed."

My arm started to get very swollen in late December. I spoke to my husband about it and he thought it might be a calcium build-up. I went back to Dr. Kendall in either January or February for my three-month checkup. After he examined me, he made no mention of my arm being swollen so I assumed it was all in my mind. This went on until March, when I noticed it was getting larger and more painful. Several of my friends noticed how I was favoring it.

I called Dr. Sloan because of the pain. He saw me that day.

Dr. Sloan came into the examining room and looked at my chart and said, "Oh yes, you're the one who is so worried about cancer." His attitude changed when he looked at my arm. He decided to take some x-rays. After looking at the films he confirmed that there was a problem.

He then went back into his office to call Dr. Kendall and didn't bother to close the door. I could hear him say, "You know that Mrs. Harnet you sent me last summer? She's in big trouble!"

His secretary told me she would set up an appointment for a bone scan and then I should see Dr. Kendall.

Exit Dr. Sloan. He was the most indifferent, uncaring physician I have ever met in my life. He was a first-class jerk.

The following Monday afternoon I had an appointment with Dr. Kendall. I told him about my conversation with Dr. Sloan and his total lack of concern. Dr. Kendall was shocked.

Dr. Kendall then recommended Dr. Andrews at Whitestone Hospital, a very fine radiologist. He was concerned before he started my radiation treatments. He wanted to have a piece of the bone analyzed to be certain the cancer was from the breast and not a new primary bone cancer.

So I had the radiation treatments to my arm. Three months later, I went to see Dr. Pesto, who took more x-rays and discovered I had another hairline fracture. He did say that these were very hard to detect. He immediately put me in a plastic brace for most of the summer. In September, to be on the safe side, he suggested I see a medical oncologist, Dr. William Dudley at St. Mary's Hospital. I went to see him in October. At that time he told us he would just watch me very closely. I would not need chemotherapy. He would do bone scans every three months. A few months later, I went for a bone scan and that is when he discovered the cancer had spread to my hip and ribs. I was immediately started on chemotherapy which I was told I would be on for a year.

I've tried to tell you as honestly and fairly as I can about the treatment I've received.

STATEMENT BY: Laura Harnet

I was watching television in my bedroom over the kitchen of our cottage when I heard a piercing scream. I ran down the stairs and found my mother bent over in pain. My father and I decided to take her over to a relative who was an orthopedic surgeon. He took a look at her, brought me into the kitchen, and said that the injury could be cancer-related because of Mom's past medical history. We all went with my mother to an emergency walk-in clinic where x-rays were taken. The radiologist said there was a slight shadow in the x-ray that was suspicious. Dr. Pesto then called Dr. Kendall to let him know what was going on. I was listening to the phone call and heard Dr. Pesto voice his opinion that the injury was cancer-related. He told me later that Dr. Kendall's reaction to his news was, "That's impossible. I saw her a few weeks ago."

The following Tuesday, Dr. Kendall admitted my mother for bone and liver scans at Whitestone Hospital.

I went to Dr. Kendall's office with Mom about six or eight months later and I remember she was still in a lot of pain and her arm was swollen and hard. The visit was very brief. He checked her chest area. He poked around her back, listened to her chest, and said she was fine. That was the end of that.

Let me make a few observations: In my mind, I felt there was something drastically wrong just by looking at her arm. It was swollen and hard. I don't think you have to be a doctor to realize there was a problem. Dr. Kendall and Dr. Sloan did not take care of my mother properly!

When Matt finished reading the statements of Mrs. Harnet and her daughter his face became flushed and he was mad! Many of their statements were outright lies. He couldn't believe what they were saying. He was crushed. Is this what medicine is all about? Who did Mrs. Harnet think he was? God? He didn't have x-ray eyes. He had called in the top bone man, who told him it was a clean break and not cancer. He had told her to come back to see him every six to eight weeks or if she noticed any change and she hadn't. When she finally got into trouble, she went to see Dr. Sloan. She was an irresponsible, bitter woman who did not listen, and he might pay the price for her ill-fated life.

"Dr. Kendall, this is Suzanne Bodman. Have you received the copies of the interrogatories taken from Mrs. Harnet and her family?"

"Yes. I've looked at them. They're a disgusting bunch of lies."

"The plaintiff's lawyers are trying to expedite a new date for trial, claiming that Mrs. Harnet is terminal. They want the case settled before she dies. I'm a little worried about this. If she gets on the stand it could have a profound effect on the jury."

"I'm sure by this time she looks like death warmed over. She's trying to say I'm responsible for her appearance, right? I gave her her cancer?"

"No, I don't think so. I think that it may be a ploy on their part. But we'd better have a defense ready, just in case they get their case moved up on the docket."

"Do you think they have a case?"

"I don't know. You can never tell what a jury will do."

"Well, I wish we could get this thing settled. It's like a cloud over my head," said Matt. "It's giving me an ulcer and making me grow old fast. It's been some time since they instituted this lawsuit. Some of my medical confreres have been asking me what happened.

"Mrs. Harnet, in her deposition, said she had continuous trouble with her arm after the fracture. I asked her how her arm was and she ignored the question. She was more interested in her facial appearance with her skin cancers. In fact, she said she was going to make an appointment to have more removed.

"The interesting part of her problem is that when she did develop recurrence of her cancer, it was a solitary recurrence at the site of the fractured arm and not a diffuse dissemination to other bones. I was the one who recommended she have a needle biopsy to determine her diagnosis. I also talked to Pesto and recommended that a medical oncologist see her and start her on chemotherapy. He recommended a medical oncologist from St. Mary's Hospital where he worked, a Dr. William Dudley.

"Radiation treatment to the solitary bone area was decided on and chemotherapy was not given by Dr. Dudley. I was sort of surprised at that, since metastatic breast cancer to the arm had been established. She should have had chemotherapy. If anyone delayed her treatment, it was the medical oncologist at St. Mary's."

"Your comments to me concerning the case have been very revealing," said Bodman. "Unfortunately, it's going to be your word against theirs. The fact that you immediately worked the patient up for spread of her cancer when she broke her arm is in your favor. Also, you did have to rely on the bone specialist for his judgment call.

"But we do have a problem. The plaintiff has given us the name of one of the leading breast cancer specialists in the country from New York City as their expert, a Dr. Harvey Jergenson. We'll have to get some other prominent cancer specialist to defend you. Do you have any suggestions?"

"Oh, God! I'm in big trouble. Harvey Jergenson is one of the leading breast cancer surgeons in the world."

"The battle is just beginning," replied Bodman. "I'm sure you must know some other comparable bigshot."

"There's a professor at Harvard who's an internationally known surgical oncologist. He might do it," said Matt. "His name is Dr. Scott Brady."

"I'll contact him and see if he'll review the case," said Bodman.

Two weeks later, Matt was informed that a deposition of his expert witness, Dr. Brady, would take place the following week. He asked Bodman whether he could be present at the deposition and was advised against it. "That's not a good idea," said Bodman. He was told, however, that he could be present when she took the deposition of the opposition's expert witness, the professor from one of the medical schools in New York City, Dr. Jergenson.

"Just what will the plaintiff's attorney be after?" asked Matt.

"They will be trying to determine if you committed professional misconduct or displayed an unreasonable lack of skill," she said.

"Medicine has many gray areas in diagnosis and treatment. How can one determine what is right and wrong, since diagnostic and treatment methods vary all over the country?" Matt asked.

"I'll try to answer that," said Suzanne. "In medical malpractice litigation, negligence is the predominant liability. In order for a patient to recover for negligent malpractice, the patient must establish the following elements: One, the existence of the doctor's duty to the patient, usually based on the existence of the physician-patient relationship. Was the patient a true patient of the doctor and had diagnostic and treatment methods been established and used? Two, was the applicable standard of care violated by the doctor being sued? Were the professional services exercised by the doctor done with the degree of skill consistent with those practiced in the community where he worked? In other words, would your colleagues have treated the patient in the same way? Three, was the injury, pain and suffering that occurred a compensable injury. Most of all, four, was there a causal connection between the violation of the standard of care and the harm?"

"That's a mouthful. I can understand why I'm in medicine and not law. This legal jargon is hard to understand. Let me ask you a question. How many lawyers are sued for malpractice?"

"Not very many. Although the number is increasing. Doctors are better targets for malpractice than lawyers. They carry a lot of insurance, much more than lawyers, which means we can collect more if we win the case. Incidentally, the law firm for the plaintiff is claiming you instituted maltreatment."

"What's maltreatment?"

"It usually refers to treatment of the patient by a doctor such as yourself. The term signifies improper or unskillful treatment. It can result either from ignorance, neglect, or willfulness."

"They're really going after my jugular, aren't they?" said Matt.

"We may be going after theirs before this is over," she said. "I believe there's an expression—'It ain't over till it's over.' I think the Harvard professor's deposition will help us determine whether we have a good or bad case. My initial impression, from talking to him on the phone, is favorable."

"Well, Dr. Brady is one of the top cancer specialists in the country," said Matt. "I know him personally. He's a brilliant surgical oncologist. I would respect his judgment and evaluation of the case, even if I lose. Do you think this case will go to trial?"

"It depends on the opposition," said Bodman. "If they think they've got a case they might win, they'll spend the time and money or they may just drag it out, hoping to collect more money for their client with a settlement."

"Could you send me a copy of the deposition of Dr. Brady after it's done?"

"I'll be glad to."

24

THE FOLLOWING WEEK, Dr. Scott Brady drove from Boston and went
to the law office of Grayson, Cummings, Wheeler, Robinson and
Stein. He was met at the entrance to the building by Suzanne Bodman.
Impeccably dressed in a dark gray flannel suit with a maroon polka-
dot bowtie, Brady was a tall, distinguished-looking gentleman. His
eyes were bright and penetrating and when he talked his voice had a
deep resonance to it.

"Do you have any questions about the case before we go into the
deposition?" asked Bodman.

Dr. Brady thought for a minute and then replied. "I've spent some
time reviewing the chart and the interrogations. There's obvious con-
flicting testimony by the plaintiff. I'm sure you're aware of that," he
said. "I hope the deposition is not too time-consuming."

"It shouldn't be," she replied.

The two went into the law office and were escorted to the conference room. Dr. Brady sat on one side of the table with Bodman and her
assistant. The opposing lawyers for the plaintiff sat on the opposite
side. A court stenographer sat in the corner.

Brady was sworn in by the stenographer.

The examination of Dr. Brady was done by Attorney Tom Buckley.

Q. "Doctor, my name is Tom Buckley. I'm one of the attorneys
who represent Helen Harnet. I'll be asking you about her case.
Have you ever been through a deposition before?"

A. "Yes."

Q. "Good. I won't have to go over how it works. However, I'll
repeat a couple of the ground rules so we understand what's
going on. If you have any trouble understanding any of my
questions, or if I use the wrong technical term, or I use it in a

context that doesn't make sense to you, just indicate that to me and I'll try to rephrase the question. Secondly, it's important that you give us a verbal response so that Mr. Sherman, the stenographer, can record it. OK?"

A. "Yes."

Q. "If at any time, after you've answered a question, you want to go back to that question and change it later and add, delete, or modify something, you're perfectly entitled to do so, and that stays true throughout the entire deposition. All right?"

A. "Yes."

Q. "Now we just talked about some stipulations. There's one other item you will have to take care of at the end of the deposition. Mr. Sherman is going to prepare a transcript, which will be sent to you to read, and at that time you can make corrections. You will have an errata sheet you can make changes on. You will then have to sign it in the presence of a notary. OK?"

A. "Yes."

Q. "Doctor, can you go through your educational background for me, beginning with college?"

A. "I went to Williams College in Williamstown, Mass. I graduated in 1975 and attended Yale School of Medicine and graduated in 1979."

Q. "After finishing your medical school training at Yale, what course of training did you go through? What was your specialty?"

A. "I completed a surgical residency at the University of Michigan Hospital and then took a fellowship in cancer at Sloan Kettering Cancer Center in New York City. I also did research for a year at the National Cancer Institute in Washington, DC."

Q. "Just how long was your training period?"

A. "Seventeen years."

Q. "What is your title at Harvard now?"

A. "Professor of Clinical Surgery. I'm the Chief of the Surgical Oncology Program."

Q. "Doctor Brady, have you ever been sued for malpractice?"

Attorney Bodman spoke up. "I object. Dr. Brady is not the doctor being sued. Dr. Kendall is."

"I understand," said Attorney Buckley. "However, we are interested in determining the credibility of this witness, since he has been designated as the expert. If you prefer, we can wait until we go to trial to ask this question."

"You may continue with your questioning," said Bodman.

A. "Yes, said Brady."

Q. "How many times?"

A. "Two."

Q. "Has a judgment ever been ruled against you?"

A. "No."

Q. "Dr. Brady, have you read and reviewed the chart of Mrs. Helen Harnet?"

A. "Yes."

Q. "In your practice in Boston do you see and treat very many breast cancer patients?"

A. "Yes."

Q. "Have you ever seen a case like Mrs. Harnet's, where a woman has broken her arm after she had breast cancer treatment?"

A. "Yes. But not exactly the same. I've taken care of a woman with breast cancer, who was in an automobile accident, suffering multiple fractures of her ribs and arms."

Q. "What happened to that patient?"

A. "She's alive and well, eight years after her accident."

Q. "Mrs. Harnet broke her arm opening a window. That's not quite the same thing, is it?"

A. "I understand she banged on the window because she couldn't open it. I wasn't there so I can't verify what she did."

Q. "What would you do if a breast cancer patient of yours, similar to Mrs. Harnet, broke her arm and you were asked to take care of her?"

A. "I'd call in an orthopedic surgeon to evaluate and treat the fracture."

Q. "Would you do anything else?"

A. "Yes. I'd do a metastatic work-up. Bone scans, x-rays, blood studies, etcetera, to see if the fracture was related to her breast cancer."

Q. "Would you consider giving the patient chemotherapy?"

A. "Only if there was evidence of spread of cancer to her bones. In other words, she would have to have a pathologic fracture."

Q. "Have you looked at Mrs. Harnet's x-rays and bone scans?"

A. "Yes."

Q. "Would you describe what you saw?"

A. "Mrs. Harnet had a undisplaced hairline fracture of the left upper humerus. The bone scan did light up in this area. The rest of her bones were normal."

Q. "Dr. Brady, what would you say if I told you that another prominent expert witness said the hairline fracture showed evidence of cancer?"

"Objection," said Bodman. "That's hearsay. Name the expert you claim made the statement for the records or withdraw the question."

"I'll withdraw the question, since our expert has not been interrogated yet," said Attorney Buckley.

Q. "I'll change the line of questioning. Dr. Brady, have you ever seen a single fracture site of metastases from breast cancer?"

A. "I'm sure it can happen, but it's extremely rare. Usually there are diffuse metastases from breast cancer to many areas and many bones are involved; spine, ribs, skull."

Q. "What if the fracture site doesn't heal?"

A. "I would assume the bone specialist would be following that patient concerning the fracture."

Q. "Wouldn't you be following that patient also, such as Mrs. Harnet?"

A. "Yes."

Q. "How long does it take for a fractured arm to heal?"

A. "I'm not sure. That depends on the type of fracture. Two or three months probably, for a routine break. I'd consult with the bone specialist."

Q. "Was Dr. Kendall seeing this patient, Mrs. Harnet, in follow up?"

A. "I believe so. I'll have to look at his office records."

Dr. Brady sifted through the records and reviewed the office notes of Dr. Kendall.

A. "Dr. Kendall saw Mrs. Harnet in the hospital when she fractured her arm and a metastatic work-up was done; bone scan, liver scan. He saw her three weeks later and she was told she would have to be watched. She was to be seen periodically by Dr. Sloan until she healed her fracture. After that, she was to return to Dr. Kendall's office every eight weeks. However, I note in his office notes, that her last visit was 18 weeks later."

Q. "How do you account for that?"

A. "I don't know."

Q. "What do you do if a cancer patient is supposed to return for follow up and doesn't come in?"

A. "We usually send a recall card."

Q. "Was it done in this case?"

A. "I don't know. I believe it was."

Q. "What if they still don't come in?"

A. "That's the patient's responsibility. A doctor can't force a patient to return for follow-up."

Q. "When did she come back?"

A. "Eighteen weeks later, according to Dr. Kendall's office notes."

Q. "Mrs. Harnet says her arm was swollen when she saw Dr. Kendall in January. Dr. Kendall made no mention of the swelling in her arm. Should he have consulted with Dr. Sloan?"

A. "According to his office notes, she was complaining about the skin cancers on her face and not her arm. You have to go by what the patient tells you."

Q. "Dr. Brady, how often have you been an expert witness on malpractice cases?"

A. "About twenty-five times. I try to avoid malpractice cases because I feel my time can be better spent in the operating room."

Q. "Dr. Brady, do you think Dr. Kendall's follow-up of this patient conforms to the practice of caring for a breast cancer patient in this area?"

A. "Absolutely."

Q. "Can you be sure of that? Our expert feels Dr. Kendall should have ordered a biopsy of the bone when she first fractured it."

"Objection," said Attorney Bodman. "That's hearsay. You can make that statement only when your expert is under oath and is present. Besides, Dr. Kendall had to rely on his expert bone specialist, the chief of orthopedics, at his hospital. He was told it was a clean hairline fracture and not related to cancer. There was nothing to biopsy at that time."

"I'll withdraw the statement," replied Attorney Buckley.

Q. "Dr. Brady, is there any statement you would like to make before we close this deposition?" asked Attorney Buckley.

A. "Yes. This is an expensive waste of my valuable time and yours. I believe that Dr. Kendall should sue the plaintiff for instituting a frivolous lawsuit."

★   ★   ★

Matt had discussed going to the courthouse to watch the selection of the jurors with Attorney Bodman.

"I wouldn't do it if I were you," she said. "The TV and newspeople will record your presence and it will be on television and your picture will be in the papers the next day."

"Hell, it's all over the newspapers already anyway." said Matt. "I think I should show the prospective jurors and the people just what kind of man I am. I'm not hiding from anyone. I'm proud of the way I practice medicine."

"Suit yourself. I'll just tell you one thing. You're to keep your mouth closed, no matter what happens. Do you understand?"

"Yes, I do."

"There is some good news. The trial has been assigned to Judge Sara Alcort, a prominent black Superior Court Judge. She's a graduate of Smith College and Harvard Law School, and has a reputation for not tolerating nonsense. With her on the bench, I feel confident we'll have a fair trial. Since she's a female, she ought to have some understanding about breast cancer and its problems."

The next day Matt went to the Superior Court to watch the selection of jurors. A pool of one-hundred and ten jurors had been chosen from the county. They were all assembled in one of the main rooms and Judge Alcort came in promptly at 10:00 A.M. to describe how the jury selection worked to the prospective jurors.

A court officer had led the jurors in to hear the instructions. There were quite a few press people present in the room, along with spectators—some had to be sent out of the room to make room for the potential jurors.

Judge Alcort emphasized the importance of jury duty to maintain justice in the county. They were told that it was their duty to listen to the evidence and to pay attention and that it would be necessary for the plaintiff—the prosecution—to prove the crime of malpractice had been committed. The defendant was to be considered innocent unless the evidence showed he was guilty and that his medical practice did not conform to the practice of other doctors who practice in his community.

The process of selecting twelve jurors to hear Dr. Kendall's malpractice case began by having the prospects fill out a questionnaire. The questionnaire required yes or no answers in most cases, a few multiple choice selections, and two questions that required essay answers. The questions concentrated on the prospective jurors opinions about pre-trial publicity, the nature of the medical case and opinions about doctors in general.

Judge Alcort released a blank copy of the questionnaire to the press. Some of the questions were routine, others could be considered controversial.

Attorney Bodman told Matt that many of the prospective jurors would be dismissed because of bias in their answers.

Thirty-nine of the prospective jurors had requested that they be excused—they had to state in writing their reasons. The lawyers from both sides reviewed the reasons and thirty-eight jurors had valid excuses not to serve on the jury. Some of the reasons were: care of sick members of their family: inability to find a replacement at work in a small company: taking medication that could impair their judgment.

One of the jurors was not excused. She was the wife of a physician. Bodman wanted to question that one herself. She was probably an intellectual and Bodman felt she wanted to get as many women and intellectuals on the jury as possible.

The prosecution interrogated the physician's wife first.

"Have you ever heard your husband talk about breast cancer?"

"Yes. Every woman knows all about it these days. It's all over the TV and radio on the talk shows."

"Have you ever had a friend or relative die from breast cancer?"

"Yes. I had a sister who died from breast cancer."

"I have no further questions," said Attorney Davis.

The prosecution specified assent for her to be selected. It was now Attorney Bodman's turn.

"Did your sister die suddenly or was it a prolonged process with pain?"

"Her cancer spread all over her body."

"How long did she have breast cancer?"

"Seven years."

"How long did she live once it spread?"

"One year."

Bodman agreed that the physician's wife should be added to the jury. She would be able to understand just what was going on in their case and would be an intelligent juror.

After seven jurors had been selected and thirty dismissed because of bias and potential negative attitudes towards doctors, Judge Alcort asked the prosecution and the defense to approach the bench.

"Attorney Bodman, you are being too selective and demanding of potential jurors. Try not to ask as many questions. Almost two weeks have gone by and we only have seven jurors."

Bodman was stunned by that statement. She had to challenge it.

"Your Honor, it's extremely important that we make sure that the prospective juror has not been prejudiced by the media coverage in this case. My client's reputation is at stake. It could become necessary for me to ask for a change of venue."

"Are you asking for that?"

"No."

"Then don't bring it up!"

It had been a long, drawn out day. Judge Alcort hit the gavel. "This court is recessed until 10 A.M. tomorrow."

As Matt walked out of the courtroom a reporter from the local TV station tried to stop him to ask him a question.

"Dr. Kendall. Dr. Kendall. Do you think you will win this case?"

"No comment," replied Matt. "My lawyer has instructed me not to answer any questions."

"What about the poor lady who's dying?"

Matt wanted to punch the reporter, but thought better of it. He had tried his best to save his patient's life. The reporter's question obviously reflected some of the spectator's opinions. He hoped the jury didn't feel that way. How did he ever get himself into this mess, anyway?

The next day Judge Alcort seemed to be intolerant of excessive questioning. Five more jurors were needed and the lawyers had made little progress.

The clerk drew the names to fill the jury box. Attorney Bodman flipped through her questionnaire lists to see if there were some that she would fight to exclude.

That afternoon a black medical technician, a hispanic banker, and a childcare faculty supervisor were selected and agreed upon. The next morning two remaining jurors were picked. There was a total of seven women and five men on the jury.

It took two weeks to select the jurors for the trial.

Taking two weeks to select the jurors made Matt extremely apprehensive. He was also worried about Dr. Jergenson's testimony. He decided to call Attorney Bodman.

"Suzanne, this is Matt Kendall. I'm worried about Jergenson. If the prosecution gets him on the stand, we'll be in big trouble."

"I'm surprised at you," said Bodman. "You're a well-known surgeon. You're supposed to have confidence and willingness to enter the arena. You sound like a wimp! We have just as good, if not a better, expert witness on our side. What we have here is a battle between two giants of medicine in a legal arena. Our expert from Boston is just as good as theirs from New York."

"Well, I'm sure glad you have that attitude," said Matt. "I felt sick to my stomach when I first heard that Dr. Jergenson was going to be their expert."

"You have to have more confidence in me," she said. "Our law firm has researched all of his books, research papers, and even looked into his family life. We have extensive information about Dr. Jergenson. We'll be ready for him when they put him on the stand.

"Incidentally, the jury is set and Attorney Ricardo Davis will be presenting their case against you tomorrow. The husband and daughter will be testifying. I've also been told they are going to show a videotape of Mrs. Harnet. They plan a big production. It should be gruesome. The beginning of the trial will make you look bad. You might think we're losing, but I assure you when it's all over and the votes are counted, we'll win!"

"Thanks," said Matt. "I've probably been reading too many local newspapers. You can understand my anxiety, I'm sure."

"Yes, I can. In fact, I don't think you should be around during the start of the trial."

The next day Laura Harnet was sworn in. "Do you swear to tell the truth, the whole truth, and nothing but the truth, so help you God?"

"I do," she replied.

A senior trial lawyer from the prosecution, Attorney Ricardo Davis, began the questioning.

"Laura, please tell the jury what happened when your mother broke her left arm."

Before she could answer, Bodman interrupted and said, "Your Honor, our law firm has taken testimony from this witness in a deposition. We believe her testimony is prejudiced, given her relationship to the plaintiff. We are willing to allow the record of the deposition to be part of the record."

"Your Honor, this is an attempt by the defense to prevent the jury from hearing the daughter's testimony," said Attorney Davis.

"I agree. Objection overruled. Proceed with the questioning," said Judge Alcort.

"Laura, please tell the jury what happened to your mother when she fractured her arm."

"I'll try, but it's going to be difficult."

In a slow, hesitating voice, she described what happened to her mother. Her histrionics, embellished with her tears could have won an academy award. She went into intimate gruesome details, elucidating all the times she took her mother to see Dr. Sloan and Dr. Kendall—describing the pain and agony her mother had to tolerate.

"Laura, did you accompany your mother when she went to see Dr. Kendall, six months after the accident?"

"Yes. My mother had swelling of her arm. She complained about it to Dr. Kendall. He seemed to ignore it."

"When did your mother realize she had spread of her cancer to her arm?"

"It was in April, I believe. She went back to see Dr. Sloan because of pain and swelling. He took some more x-rays and found the cancer had spread. She overheard him call Dr. Kendall and tell him that she was in big trouble."

"I have no further questions, Your Honor."

"Attorney Bodman, your witness."

"Laura, when you went to Dr. Kendall's office with your mother, did you go back in the examining room with her or did she go alone?"

"I don't remember," she replied.

"Your Honor, I believe the witness should have to answer. She seems to remember every other detail."

"Answer yes or no," said Judge Alcort.

"No," she replied.

"Laura, in Dr. Kendall's office after your mother was seen, was she given a card giving the date and time of her next appointment before she left his office?"

"Your Honor, I have to object to this line of questioning," said Attorney Davis. "What relevance does this have to the suit against Dr. Kendall?"

"Your Honor, it's completely relevant. The prosecution claims there was delay in diagnosis and treatment of Mrs. Harnet. She was told and was given an appointment to come in every eight weeks so she could be watched. An appointment card was given to her. She chose to come back 18 weeks later. Laura Harnet was given that appointment card for her mother's appointment."

"Objection overruled."

"I did receive that card," said Laura.

"No further questions, Your Honor," said Bodman, as she sat down.

The next morning at 10:00 A.M. the case resumed with Attorney Davis asking further questions.

"Your Honor . . . as you know, my client, Mrs. Harnet, is too sick to come to this courthouse to present her side of the story. We have recently made a video so that the jury can see what she looks like. We have also asked her to answer a few pertinent questions."

"Objection!" said Bodman. "How am I going to question Mrs. Harnet if she's on a video?"

"We've asked her just to answer a few simple questions," replied Davis.

"I object, Your Honor!" repeated Bodman. "This is a ploy on Attorney Davis' part to prejudice the jury."

"It is not!" said Davis, as his neck started to get red above his collar.

"If you show that video," said Bodman, "I want to remind the jury that Dr. Kendall did not operate on Mrs. Harnet's right breast. It was botched up by another surgeon! We'll admit that he did remove her left breast for cancer, and by doing so saved her life. My client is not responsible for what she looks like now!"

"That's exactly where we differ!" shouted Davis. "If Dr. Kendall had practiced judicious judgement and diagnosed Mrs. Harnet's cancer earlier, she wouldn't look the way she does now."

Bodman shouted right back at Davis. "Your Honor! That statement by Attorney Davis should be stricken from the record. It has not been proven that Dr. Kendall used poor judgement in the management of Mrs. Harnet's case!"

Judge Alcort banged her gavel. "Calm down!" she said. "That statement will be removed from the record. The jury is to ignore that last statement. However, Attorney Bodman, your objection to showing the video is overruled. If I feel the questioning on the video is prejudiced, the video will be withdrawn from the evidence."

"Thank you, Your Honor," replied Bodman.

The video was then shown and had an obvious effect on the jury. Mrs. Harnet was a very sick emaciated woman dying from cancer. After the showing of the video, Judge Alcort banged her gavel. "That will be all for today. Court will resume at 10:00 A.M. tomorrow."

That evening the late edition of the *Whitestone Times* had complete verbatim coverage of the debate between Attorney Davis and Attorney Bodman about the showing of the video to the jury. It was also on the 6:00 TV news.

The next day, court was called back into session. The courtroom was packed because of the newspaper and media coverage.

"Call Dr. Harvey Jergenson to the stand," said Attorney Davis.

"Do you swear to tell the truth, the whole truth and nothing but the truth, so help you God?"

The professor took the stand. "I do."

"Dr. Jergenson, you have an extensive training background, many honorary degrees, published books on breast disease, have done research in this field, and headed a department of surgery. Have you reviewed the chart and records on Mrs. Harnet?"

"I have."

"If you were taking care of Mrs. Harnet when she fractured her arm, what would you have done?"

"I would have done an extensive work-up to rule out spread of her cancer."

"What tests would you do?"

"I'd do radioactive scans of the bones and liver or a CAT scan or MRI to see if the tissues were normal."

"Would you do anything else?"

"I'd do a needle biopsy of the fracture site if it didn't look right. I'd try to get a piece of tissue to see if cancer was present."

"What if the tests were all negative? Is there anything else you would do?"

"I'd tell that patient she would have to see me frequently and that she would have to undergo further testing if she developed any symptoms."

"Were all these tests done on Mrs. Harnet?"

"No," replied Dr. Jergenson. "The bone biopsy was not done."

"Is there anything else that you would have done?"

"I would have repeated all of her tests six months after the date of her fracture."

"Was that done?"

"I believe that Dr. Sloan did x-ray her arm four months after her fracture."

"Were any other tests done?"

"No," replied Dr. Jergenson. "I believe Dr. Kendall did not repeat any of her x-ray tests after that until her cancer had metastasized. There definitely was delay in diagnosis."

"I have no further questions, Your Honor."

"Your witness," said Judge Alcort, as she leaned forward in her chair, looking on in interest as the medical heavyweights slugged it out.

"Dr. Jergenson, did Mrs. Harnet have radioactive scans of her liver and bones or CAT scans to rule out spread of her cancer when she fractured her arm?" Bodman smiled as she spoke.

"I believe so."

"Please answer yes or no."

"Yes."

"Have you seen the x-rays of the fracture that Mrs. Harnet had?"

"No."

"Your Honor, I have a copy of those x-rays which I'd like to project on the screen for the jury, as well as for Dr. Jergenson."

"Your Honor, I object to Attorney Bodman's line of questioning. Dr. Jergenson is not the doctor who took care of Mrs. Harnet," said Attorney Davis. "He's not the doctor on trial. His judgement is germane only insofar as it pertains to his experience with this type of case."

"Judge Alcort, I wish to show the x-rays to Dr. Jergenson so he can tell us just where he would biopsy the fracture Mrs. Harnet sustained. After all, he's the expert in this field. He testified that he would have done a bone biopsy when she first fractured her arm."

"Objection overruled."

The x-rays of Mrs. Harnet were projected on the large screen for the jury to see.

"Dr. Jergenson, what do you see on those x-rays?"

"I see a fracture of the left upper arm."

"Would you point it out with the pointer?"

Dr. Jergenson was given a pointer. He walked to the screen and pointed to the middle of the left upper arm.

"I don't see what you're pointing at," said Bodman.

"It's hard to see," said Dr. Jergenson, squinting.

"The first x-rays are exhibit A," said Attorney Bodman. "We have some other x-rays to show."

The projectionist put up more x-rays on the screen, showing another aspect of the left arm.

"What do you see in these x-rays?"

"I think I see a small fracture of the left upper arm."

"Where would you biopsy that arm?"

"It's hard to tell," said Dr. Jergenson. "Probably in the middle of the shaft of the bone, like the other one. Right here," he said as he used the pointer.

"Aren't you supposed to biopsy the fracture site?" asked Attorney Bodman.

"That's correct," said Dr. Jergenson. "That's the fracture site."

"The second x-rays are exhibit B," said Attorney Bodman. "Dr. Jergenson, have you ever been sued for malpractice?"

"I object, Your Honor," said Attorney Davis. "Dr. Jergenson is not on trial here."

"Your Honor, I'm trying to determine the credibility of this expert witness."

"You may continue. Objection overruled."

"Well, have you been sued?"

"Yes."

"How many times?"

"Any good doctor is sued for malpractice these days."

"Please answer the question yes or no."

"Yes. As director of a surgical teaching department in a large university hospital, I've been sued frequently, since I have to defend the young doctors training under me."

"How many times, Dr. Jergenson?"

"Eight."

"How many verdicts have been ruled against you or your students?"

"Three times," said Dr. Jergenson. "The residents made the mistakes. Not me."

"Were you present at the operations?" asked Bodman.

"Yes."

"Dr. Jergenson, how many operations do you do a week?"

"You mean now or when I was busy?"

"I mean right now or during the past year," replied Bodman.

"I'm an emeritus professor. I'm not operating any more."

"How long has it been since you were in an operating room?"

"Five years."

"How old are you?"

"Seventy-six years old."

"Have you done any stereotaxic biopsies of the breast?"

"I don't understand. What do you mean? Will you rephrase the question?"

"I'll repeat the question. Have you done any stereotaxic biopsies of the breast?"

"I'm sorry. I can't answer that question. I don't know what you mean."

"Your Honor, I'd like to ask for a recess to talk to my witness," said Attorney Davis.

Judge Alcort banged the gavel down. "Recess granted. We'll reconvene in the morning with Dr. Jergenson as the witness."

25

THAT EVENING, Dr. Kendall received a call at home from Suzanne Bodman.

"Matt, Mrs. Harnet's lawyers would like to settle the case."

"My God. What happened?"

"The trial went very well today. I think we destroyed Jergenson as an expert witness. He hasn't practiced surgery for five years and was unable to answer a key question. He didn't know what a stereotaxic biopsy was. I don't either, for that matter. Dr. Brady suggested that question. I understand it's a new breast x-ray biopsy technique. His failure to answer that question shows that he has not kept up with current breast diagnostic methods."

"When he testified that he would have biopsied the fracture site when Mrs. Harnet broke her arm, I showed him two x-rays and asked him where he would biopsy the hairline fracture site. The second x-ray he pointed to for a biopsy was a normal x-ray. He didn't know that. I plan to bring that point out tomorrow. We do have a problem, however, and you will have to make the ultimate decision."

"What's the problem?" asked Matt.

"The prosecution called and said that they will drop the case against you completely, if you will sign a paper stating you will not sue them for instituting a frivolous lawsuit."

"You've got to be kidding. After all I've gone through and all my family has gone through the past three years?"

"I think you should do it. Give it some serious thought. Talk to your wife. You have till tomorrow morning at nine o'clock to make the decision."

Matt's immediate reaction was profound elation and relief. He was free at last. His lawyer had done a brilliant job in defending him. She had proven he had not committed malpractice, or had she? However, the acute and chronic stress had taken its toll. The lines in his face had deepened, his hair had gotten thinner and gray, and his ego had been shattered. He was angry and disgusted by what had happened.

"I'm not going to sign the papers! They're a bunch of bastards!" he hollered. "I'm going to sue them for their eye teeth. I've been through hell! Their actions have permanently damaged my professional reputation."

"I think we have to sit down and talk about this," said Nancy. "If you did sue them, it would take another three years before it came to trial and you'd still be under severe stress. You might not live through it. What would you gain?"

"Peace of mind. They instituted a frivolous lawsuit against me so they could get rich. They shouldn't be able to get off the hook that easily."

"Perhaps we should, as the Bible advises, turn the other cheek," said Nancy.

Matt hollered harshly, "Don't give me that! They started it. It also says in that book, 'An eye for an eye, a tooth for a tooth.' They practically destroyed me as a surgeon, mentally, physically, and economically."

"You still haven't answered my question. What have you to gain by suing the family of a patient who's dying of breast cancer?"

"I'd educate the public," replied Matt. "Medical decisions are complex and there is a common and mistaken assumption that doctors can simply process all relevant information and arrive at correct answers. Medicine is not an exact science. I kept that lady alive for over five years. She was an extremely difficult patient to take care of and she did not cooperate or communicate."

"Think for a minute," said Nancy. "If you have a new trial the news media may not give you proper publicity. Doctors are not as popular as they used to be. You won't get the newspaper headlines like when you were first sued. It'll end up on the back page, in the bottom corner, where no one will even notice. We have to make the proper decision and just sign the papers, Honey. We don't have a lot of time. What's the advice of your lawyer?"

"She said I ought to sign. It would be just another prolonged headache if I didn't."

"I think she's right. Why don't you call your brother? After all, he's a Superior Court Judge. He should be able to give you some advice."

"That's not a bad idea. I'll call him right away."

Matt dialed the phone and got his brother Mark.

"Mark, Matt. I've got a problem and I want you to tell me how I should resolve it."

"You're not having another fight with your wife, are you?"

"Just a disagreement. I want to talk to you about my malpractice case. You've probably read in the papers that the trial has started."

"Yes, I did. How's it going?"

"OK, so far."

"You've got a good lawyer defending you. Bodman has an excellent reputation. I've heard a few of her cases in my courtroom."

"Well, that's why I called. She's a terrific lawyer. She called me today and told me the prosecution wants to drop the case."

"That's great! You can start living a normal life again."

"It's not that simple. The prosecution wants me to sign a paper stating I won't sue their client for instituting a frivolous lawsuit."

"I'd sign it."

"If I sign it, I'm admitting I'm guilty."

"No, you're not! They're asking you to give up something so they won't proceed with the prosecution of your case. Evidentally, they feel the jury may vote in your favor and they may lose the case. They want to reach a settlement."

"But that's letting the prosecution get away with instituting a malpractice suit that shouldn't have taken place."

"In law, you find out there's two sides to every question. It's the interpretation of the law that determines whether someone is guilty or innocent. No one knows how that jury will decide. If the prosecution drops the case, the jury will not be given the opportunity to vote. Don't forget that! I'd sign it."

"Thanks for your advice."

Matt decided to sign and put an end to the malpractice case against him once and for all.

26

NOW THAT THE trial in Superior Court was over, Nancy thanked God for the withdrawal of the lawsuit against her husband. She called her children who were scattered around the country in Lancaster, Jacksonville, Atlanta, and Philadelphia, and told them the good news.

Three years of acute and chronic stress had taken a lot out of her and Matt.

Matt's main problem during the trial was that he was having difficulty rationalizing why he was being sued. He felt he had done nothing wrong and Nancy agreed with him.

"Every good doctor gets sued, particularly if he takes risks to save someone's life," said Nancy. "Our country has a litigious society. There are too many lawyers who are looking for a fast buck!"

"The public doesn't know what's going on," said Matt. "It's too bad they're not better informed."

"I blame the media for that—also our complacent elected officials," said Nancy.

"Most of us, as we go through life, hope it's a pleasant experience. However, everyone eventually dies. What happens shouldn't end up in the courthouse."

A week before Labor Day, as he was driving home, Matt called Nancy from his car phone. "Do you want to eat at home or do you want to go out tonight?"

"I don't feel like cooking. Why don't you stop at Gino's and bring home a pizza."

"OK," replied Matt.

When they finished the pizza Nancy said, "I'm going to the mall and pick up a couple of new blouses. Mike is flying up from Jacksonville next week for a visit and I want to look nice."

"Fine. I'll watch Monday night football."

When Nancy got home from the mall Matt noticed that she looked sick—a big change from the way she looked at dinner time.

"What happened to you?" he asked.

"I think I caught a bug. I had shaking chills while I was shopping."

"We'd better take your temperature. Do you have any belly pain? Has anyone been sick at work?"

"No one that I know of. I do have a little discomfort in my right upper abdomen, though, and a stiff neck."

"Do you have a sore throat?"

"No," she replied. "But I ache all over."

Matt got a thermometer and placed it in Nancy's mouth.

"104°. Wow! You really are burning up!"

Matt was worried about meningitis (a lethal bacterial infection that involves the brain)—a stiff neck is one of the symptoms.

"We'd better start you on an antibiotic. Do we have any?"

"I think I have some Amoxicillin in the cupboard."

"Should we call your doctor?"

"No. I think I must have a flu bug. I'll go to bed and try to sleep it off."

Matt didn't fall asleep and Nancy was restless, tossing and turning. Matt's medical-surgical mind started to dream up all sorts of calamitous situations.

At 2 A.M. he asked her how she felt.

"I haven't slept a wink and I still feel horrible."

He took her temperature and it was 102°.

"Your temp has come down a little. Drink some more ice water and take some Tylenol."

Matt was beginning to worry about what the next day would bring and how she would feel. He was operating in the morning and would have to leave for the hospital.

Six A.M. seemed to arrive all too fast. He took her temperature. It was 101°. He was really worried about leaving her alone.

"What do you think we should do?" he asked.

"I think I'll be all right. I'll call your office if I feel worse."

He decided to call his secretary, Judy, to let her know what was going on. He asked her to call and check on Nancy periodically while he was in the operating room.

"My wife's a stoic, you know. You have to pry to get any information out of her."

"I understand," replied Judy. "Hopefully, she just has the flu."

Matt had a full surgery schedule. He cancelled out as much of his afternoon office patients as he could and arrived home at 5 P.M.

"I feel a little better," said Nancy. "I'm sure it's only a flu bug." She tried to be reassuring, although her voice was tremulous.

"You don't look any better. If you're not better by tomorrow I'm taking you to have some blood work done. I'll have you see Dr. Fern, the surgeon who covers me when I'm away."

The next morning, she wasn't any better and he took her in to the blood lab and had them do blood cultures, a complete blood count and a Chem 24—computerized blood test that checks liver and kidney functions. He told the girl drawing the blood to *stat* the blood work so they could get the results as soon as possible.

Dr. Fern examined Nancy and ordered an ultrasound of her gall-bladder and pancreas and flat plate x-rays of her abdomen and chest.

The girl in the lab forgot to stat the blood work so the results were unavailable until that evening.

When the results were finally obtained, there was no elevation of her white blood count—it was 6500. However, her platelets, which take part in the clotting mechanism of blood, were down somewhat, suggesting a possible virus infection.

Dr. Fern called to say her x-rays were all normal. "No gallstones, no pancreatic abnormalities, normal bowel x-rays, and her chest is clear."

"What do you think is going on?"

"I think she has an acute viral infection and needs to see an infectious disease specialist."

"Who's available?"

"Dr. Herbert Jones, one of the younger men. He's good."

"Give him a call and set up an appointment."

The next morning, Matt took Nancy to see Dr. Jones.

He took an extensive history, did a physical exam, and finally came out into the room where Matt was waiting.

"I've ordered some more blood work on your wife. I think she has a viral infection—somewhat like the flu. It may be just a transitory thing. If she gets worse give me a call."

Matt thought about that. She *was* worse! He was a surgeon and when he saw patients, he usually operated on them to find out what was wrong. He had opened many bellies to drain abscesses or remove an appendix. Now he had to wait expectantly—almost like waiting for his wife to have a baby—hoping and praying she would be all right. The shoe was on the other foot now. He wasn't making the decisions and he didn't like it. He remembered when he was an intern and how he hated medicine because of the inaction. That's why he had become a surgeon. He wanted answers.

"Are you absolutely sure she has a viral infection?"

"I'm not one hundred percent sure. That's why I ordered more blood work." Dr. Jones then repeated, "If she gets worse call me."

Matt looked at Dr. Jones in amazement. He decided to say nothing.

There were beads of sweat on Matt's forehead as he took Nancy's hand and they left Dr. Jones' office. Nancy dragged her feet as she walked to the parking lot.

As he got the car out onto the highway, Nancy looked taut and apprehensive and spoke up, "I think I have to vomit. I can't control it. I feel awfully sick. I've never felt like this before."

Suddenly she erupted, vomiting all over the dashboard.

Matt decided to take her directly to the hospital and called Dr. Jones from his car phone.

After Nancy was admitted, she was placed in a bed in the medical intensive care unit.

The nurse took her temp. It was 104°. Her pulse was 110 and her blood pressure was 85/50.

"Do you usually have a low blood pressure?" asked the nurse.

"I do a lot of walking. My pressure is usually 100/70," Nancy replied. "Why do you ask?"

"I just wanted to know."

The nurse quickly walked out of the room and called Dr. Jones.

"That patient you just admitted, Mrs. Kendall, looks very sick. Her temp is 104°, pulse is rapid, blood pressure is down to 85/50. She looks dehydrated and states she's been vomiting."

"Get the IV team up there stat and start some intravenous saline. We don't have her blood work back yet. I also want to start her on some intravenous antibiotics just in case this isn't a virus infection."

"I don't like her low blood pressure," said the nurse, expressing her concern.

"I don't either!" said Dr. Jones. "Put her on hourly vital signs. I'll call the lab and see if her blood work is ready. Also give her Tylenol for that temp. She could be going into septic shock."

Matt decided to stay at the hospital with Nancy that evening.

"I feel awful, Matt. I think you'd better notify the children. I'm not sure I'm going to make it."

Nancy's comment and concern made him feel like he'd been kicked in the stomach. Tears came to his eyes. Nancy had always been strong, never sick. Now she was deathly ill, fighting for her life, and her doctors didn't know what was going on or what to do for her. He felt helpless.

"Go make the calls. Please, do it for me."

"I will, Honey," responded Matt.

He made four long-distance calls, starting with the oldest and ending with the youngest.

He called Betsy first. She was married to a general practitioner in Lancaster, Pennsylvania and they had three children.

Next, he called Mike, a gastroenterologist, living in Jacksonville, Florida. He was very concerned about his mother and said he would catch the next plane.

Matt then called Susan, a nurse living in Atlanta, Georgia, married to a minister with a one-year-old boy.

The youngest, Karen, was a paralegal working in Philadelphia. After hearing about her mother, she decided to drive up to see her.

After making the phone calls, Matt went back to Nancy's room. Dr. Jones was there examining her. He had a frown on his brow and looked troubled as he came out of the room.

"Your wife's got a serious infection," he said. "Her white blood count and her platelet count keep going down. Her liver studies are also abnormal."

"What can we do?"

"We don't have any good medicines for viruses and it looks like that's what she's got. Viruses can be lethal. All you can do is treat the patient symptomatically."

"Why are her liver chemistries out of whack?"

"Because the virus is attacking her liver."

"Should we still be giving antibiotics if she's got a virus infection? Won't the antibiotics make the virus worse?"

"No. A serious bacterial infection can sometimes give you the same blood picture. That's why we're still giving her high-dose antibiotics."

"Could she have Lyme Disease or Legionnaires' Disease?"

"All those tests are in the works but it doesn't look like she does."

"Is there anything else we can do? Should we get another opinion?"

"If her blood picture gets worse, I'll call a hematologist in to advise us," said Dr. Jones.

"I'd call him in now," said Matt. "We need all the help we can get! God, she looks so sick lying there flat on the bed with her eyes closed."

When Karen arrived from Philadelphia, she was shocked when she saw how sick her mother was.

"Can't they do something, Dad?"

"I guess not. They really don't know what's going on. They think she's got a virus infection but they're not sure."

"Could they be missing something? Is there something I can do to help Mom?"

"Yes, there is," said Matt. "She's not eating. She's only drinking sips of water and getting intravenous fluids. Your brother wants her to try to drink some Gatorade."

More blood was drawn from Nancy's arms for blood cultures, blood counts, and liver and kidney studies. Her urine and stools were also cultured. All the blood culture reports were negative. She continued to get worse. Her immune system was going into failure. Her white count was down to 3000 and her platelets were down to 33,000. Her red cells were also down. Her hematocrit, which measures red cells, was 27 and falling.

Dr. Jones was also obviously getting more concerned. He called in Dr. Stewart, a specialist in blood disease.

"Just what is happening?" Matt asked Dr. Stewart.

"The virus is attacking her bone marrow. That's where all her blood is made. What's scary is that her platelet count is still going down and she's not making any red cells. Without platelets, she won't be able to clot her blood and she needs her red cells to carry oxygen to the tissues. She could develop an uncontrollable hemorrhage."

On Saturday, Nancy seemed to be slipping away. She was no longer mentally alert. Matt was pacing the hall outside her room. Karen remained in the room, watching her mother. At 2 P.M. Karen came and told him that Nancy was getting worse. Her respiratory rate had suddenly increased to 34, her pulse was irregular, and she was having difficulty breathing. She told Karen she was breathless.

Matt called the assistant head nurse and told her he wanted Dr. Jones called immediately. He also told the nurse that he wanted a stat chest x-ray done on his wife.

"I'll have to call Dr. Jones first and get his permission."

"Do what you want, but I want that x-ray done!"

Nancy was taken down to the x-ray department on a stretcher and Matt accompanied her.

They took two pictures of Nancy's chest. One of the senior radiologists, Dr. Gibbons, looked at her films and told Matt that she had an interstitial viral pneumonia. She had fluid in both lungs.

"Are you sure?" asked Matt.

"As sure as I can be," he replied.

Matt asked another radiologist, Dr. Fine, to look at the films.

"I think your wife has a fluid overload," said the young radiologist. "I don't think it's a viral pneumonia."

"That's great! I think we'd better get a cardiologist in to see her. We may even need to get a referee to decide what she really has!"

Matt called Dr. Jones and suggested he get a cardiologist to see Nancy. "Get Dr. Gambino to see her. He does all the consults on my pre-op surgical patients."

Dr. Gambino spent a long time checking Nancy. He looked at her chest x-ray and electrocardiogram and agreed that she had a fluid overload—10,000 cc. of fluid in three days—too much in too short a time.

"Matt, all your wife needs is a good diuretic like Lasix and she'll get rid of all that water in her lungs. I'm also going to order an echocardiogram to check her heart muscle and valves. Sometimes a virus attacks the heart. I don't like that low blood pressure, though. That virus she's got is a bad one!"

Saturday night was a bad one for Nancy, even though her echocardiogram was negative.

Mike had to fly back to Jacksonville the next day and was not happy about leaving.

Matt was losing his composure. He was frustrated by the inaction. Nancy was lying flat in a hospital bed, desperately ill, her eyes closed, her skin a dark ashen color, fighting for her life. There were intravenous tubes attached to her arms and nasal oxygen was being pumped to help ease her breathing.

The stress of her mother's illness was beginning to show on Karen, too. She decided to stay to help her mother and give her dad support. She encouraged her mother to drink, eat, and to relax as she read to her while she lay in bed.

Nancy continued to spike her temp to 104° and the shivering and teeth chattering continued. She started to complain about seeing spots and images in front of her eyes when her eyelids were closed.

Dr. Jones made a late Saturday night visit because he was concerned. Nancy was now listed as critical.

The next morning, Nancy was spoon-fed by Karen and managed to eat a little warm oatmeal. She looked like she was getting slightly better but it was only a façade. Nancy knew that Mike had to leave and fly back to Jacksonville. She didn't want him to leave because she was afraid she might not see him again. She had tears in her eyes as he said goodbye and cried openly after he left.

The next day, Nancy had a relapse, with continuing shaking chills and teeth chattering. Her blood pressure started to drop again into the eighties and she stopped eating. She was given almost all her fluids by intravenous now and only took sips of water by mouth.

She had a new symptom, a facial tic that was quite noticeable—a muscle in her cheek twitched involuntarily. She continued to complain about seeing spots and eerie peculiar shapes beneath her eyelids. Her vision was also impaired. She couldn't read or see well with her glasses. When she opened her eyes, the lights seemed very bright to her and the bright colors bothered her eyes.

Her liver chemistries (blood tests) had gotten worse. Her LDH and transaminase tests were very high, indicating that the virus was damaging her liver tissues. An ultrasound showed that her liver was enlarging and was taking up more of her abdomen. Her flat belly was now protuberant. Nancy noticed this herself and pointed it out to Matt.

Another development occurred. Blood tests that are used to check the pancreas became abnormal. Her lipase and serum amalase were elevated, suggesting that the virus was also attacking her pancreas.

What's next? What a horrible predicament! thought Matt. It looked like the virus was hitting all of her organs—liver, pancreas, and even her brain.

★　★　★

Matt discussed Nancy's eye signs with an ophthalmologist. He felt that she may need a spinal tap or a CAT scan. The ophthalmologist frightened Matt when he told him that Nancy's optic nerves were swollen and that some viruses can attack the retina and the optic nerve and cause blindness.

It looked like Nancy was losing the battle. She seemed to be losing her will to live and asked Matt to have the family minister see her. Everyone at the church was praying for her. Matt kept saying prayers and was getting exasperated because they didn't seem to be working.

"God! Why hast thou forsaken me?" he asked.

The next afternoon, Dr. Fern, came in to pay a visit. While examining Nancy's abdomen, he noted that she had a fine rash on her belly.

Matt hadn't seen very many rashes. He thought Nancy was getting meningitis and was worried because she was no longer on antibiotics.

The rash was extremely worrisome to him, but not to the young infectious disease specialist, Dr. Jones. After looking at Nancy's belly, he came out of her room and calmly announced, "I think your wife is going to get better now."

"Why do you say that?"

"Because the rash suggests that she is now making antibodies against the virus. It's like measles in kids. When they get the rash, they start to get better."

Sure enough, the next morning Nancy's temperature returned to normal. She was sitting up in bed, her eyes were open, and she started to eat. She had oatmeal and fruit for breakfast.

There were tears in Matt's and Karen's eyes when they saw her sitting up in bed for the first time.

Her temp stayed down during the next two days. She began to eat better as her blood picture improved and she was finally discharged.

During Nancy's six-week rehabilitation, she and Matt had many long discussions about the past and future.

"I guess I must have been pretty sick."

"Too close to death, as far as I'm concerned," said Matt.

"While I had all of my senses, I realized I was very sick and I prayed to God for help. I said the 23rd Psalm to myself over and over again, as far as I could remember it."

The Lord is my shepherd, I shall not want. He maketh me to lie down in green pastures. He leadth me beside the still waters. He restoreth my soul. He leadeth me in the paths of righteousness for his name's sake. Yea, though I walk through the valley of the shadow of death, I will fear no evil; for thou art with me; thy rod and thy staff they comfort me.

"Hold it right there," said Matt. "You certainly were walking through the valley of the shadow of death."

"I realize that now. I really thought I was going to die when I couldn't remember the entire 23rd Psalm. My mind started doing crazy things. That's probably when the virus started affecting my brain. That's about all I remember until I started to come out of it. My strength was my faith in God and the love I felt coming from you, Mike, and Karen."

"Well, Nancy, I'm not ready to get rid of you yet."

Matt had a smile on his face and Nancy gave him a dirty look.

She then looked him straight in the eye with a stern expression. "Matt, I think you should hang up your scalpel. You've devoted your life to taking care of patients with cancer for over thirty years. You've fought the good fight. I want to share some part of my life on earth with you, hoping to smell the roses before we are six feet under."

"Nancy, if you promise not to scare me like you did when you were sick, I'll give it serious consideration."

Matt had been in practice for over thirty years. There were so many changes rapidly developing in his field of surgery that it was mind-boggling!

Some things he liked and other's he didn't. General surgery was no longer general surgery as he had known it. In the past, he had done surgery in practically all the anatomical areas of the human body with few, if any, restrictions once he had established his reputation.

The term "general" is a misnomer now—surgery has been divided into highly specialized areas of expertise—the divisions were so numerous, it was difficult to keep up with. There are peripheral vascular surgeons; colorectal surgeons; head and neck surgeons; pediatric surgeons; hand surgeons; cardiac surgeons; thoracic surgeons; cancer surgeons; transplant surgeons; trauma surgeons; the latest group of new surgeons are laparoscopic surgeons. This great division of specialization has reduced the patient load for the general surgeons to practically zero. The age of super-specialized surgery has made a major contribution in improving some segments of healthcare but at a price.

All surgeons, including the general surgeons, have a new threat in the operating room because of the daily exposure to blood and blood products. The new threat, AIDS, is a serious one because the surgeon can't always identify the patient with AIDS. To identify the patient would be an invasion of privacy.

Other problems, such as hepatitis and new severe infections in the immune-compromised patient are also a daily risk as the surgeons continue to tackle the problems of dealing with an aging population who are sick.

The operating rooms have also enlarged and have numerous sophisticated expensive equipment for the new surgical specialties. There are lasers, argon beams, television monitors, fiberoptic scopes, stapling devices, miniaturized laparoscopic surgical instruments—all costly and frequently disposable.

In Matt's field of cancer surgery, there is a decrease in radical surgery and an increasing reliance on the team approach to treatment. Numerous disciplines are involved in the decision making—radiation and chemotherapy are being used more often.

Anesthesia has made great strides, and sophisticated anesthesia monitoring equipment is now used on all patients. Blood pressure, pulse, oxygenation of the lungs, urinary and kidney output are all monitored instantaneously and can be read on a panel as they occur.

There are also computerized laboratories available to measure changes in the blood as the surgeon operates.

The stress in the operating room, however, still remains the same— there seems to be a never-ending supply of patients who are critically ill and need surgery. Life is sustained but death often enters the surgical arena.

There is a new dress code in the operating room. All personnel have to wear expensive waterproof protective gowns, waterproof boots, and protective eyewear. The surgeons are beginning to dress more and more like the astronauts who travel in outer space.

All this fancy expensive equipment is worn to protect the personnel who work in the OR. Even if you aren't directly involved with the surgical care of the AIDS patient, you certainly know these patients are around on the operating room floor just by smelling the clorox odor in the hallways after an AIDS patient has been taken care of. Clorox is a disinfectant effective against the AIDS virus.

All that is needed to get AIDS is to have one little break in the system where the virus can break through the skin to get into the bloodstream—scalpels, needles, and surgical instruments all become contaminated with blood from AIDS patients—including the anesthesia machines.

One of the more serious accidents that happen with personnel is when an individual is inadvertently stuck with a needle used in drawing blood from an AIDS patient or when a surgeon or scrub nurse have their gloved hand or finger perforated, or "stuck," with a needle.

This happened to Matt one day when he was operating on a patient with a groin mass. The patient was a lawyer who was thought to have a lymphoma—a form of cancer. He told Matt he was a straight arrow.

Matt surgically removed the mass and gave it to the pathologist for a frozen section analysis of the tissue. The surgical resident assisting Matt wanted to close the wound so Matt let him do it. Unfortunately, the resident inadvertently stuck Matt's left forefinger with a needle—drawing blood.

"Ouch! Watch what you're doing," hollered Matt. He took his glove off and used an antiseptic on the skin break.

Matt later got the shock of his life when the pathologist came back and said, "Does this patient have AIDS?"

"Why?" Matt asked.

"Because this tissue shows florid follicular hyperplasia—often seen in AIDS patients."

"That's great!" said Matt. "I asked the patient if he practiced homosexual sex and he denied it. He's a lawyer and he lied to his doctor. He slips through the system and now I may have AIDS."

27

THE LAST BREAKFAST FOR THE INNER SANCTUM BRAIN TRUST

"WELL, GENTLEMEN, is it going to be doom and gloom today or is it going to be back to the future? Are we going to be optimistic or pessimistic?" asked Mr. Snow, chief administrator of the hospital.

"It depends on what you want to talk about," said Dr. Andrews, the general practitioner, as he looked around the room. All of the brain trust was seated around the table. The only departure from their normal meeting was white linens on the table.

"Why do we have white linen today?" asked Dr. Alford, the psychiatrist.

"Because we want to find out how many of you guys are slobs," said Bill Burns, the urologist.

"Seriously, why the pomp and circumstance?" asked Bill Milstein, the neurosurgeon.

"Because this may be the last breakfast for the Inner Sanctum Brain Trust," said Snow.

"Why?" asked Steve Walters.

"Because the Brain Trust is breaking up. Bill Burns is retiring to Arizona. Dr. Burns says he doesn't like what he sees on the horizon. He says big business and bureaucracy are destroying medicine." Snow measured his words in an awkward attempt to hide his disagreement with Burns.

"That's right," said Bill. "And you're part of that bureaucracy. When an administrator of a hospital makes twice as much as I do, that's reason enough for me to quit."

Snow's face turned red. "You're implying that I'm not worth what they're paying me?"

"Precisely. Doctors in this hospital have to spend fifteen years in training to become specialists and many don't come close to your salary. Some are lucky to make one-third of what you make."

Snow's neck was turning a deep crimson.

"Out of curiosity, Mr. Snow, just what is your educational background?" asked Andrews.

"Four years in an Ivy League school and two more years in hospital administration."

"Let's not get stuck on comparing education and salaries," said Alford, the psychiatrist. "We're all going to take a big pay cut if we get National Health Care."

"You're just jealous because you don't have a salaried job like his," Burns shot back.

"That may well be," said Alford, not willing to argue.

"Dr. Kendall's also going to be leaving us," Snow said.

"Matt, are you retiring?" asked Steve Walters.

"No. However, I am leaving medicine."

A waiter came into the doctor's dining room and started serving breakfast: eggs benedict, melon, croissants, and fresh orange juice. A cut above the donuts they were used to.

"Since this is the last breakfast of the Inner Sanctum Brain Trust, perhaps we ought to tackle some of the big problems we've been talking about for the past twenty-five years."

"I've got an agenda," said Snow. "I want to pick your brains for the last time. Also I want a question and answer period with Bill Burns and Matt Kendall answering the questions. They've each been in practice over thirty years at Whitestone Hospital and they might be willing to free-wheel-it since they're both leaving medicine. Do you mind if I tape our discussion for posterity?"

"Fire away," said Milstein. "But you might not like what you hear."

"First, I want to discuss the AIDS problems in our society and also any other infections or disease problems you guys see on the horizon."

There was a large groan from the group.

Matt was silent. He hesitated for a moment and then spoke up. "I'll open the discussion. The AIDS problem recently hit me in the face. I was operating on a lawyer, who lied to me about his past. He had been a drug abuser and bisexual and had frequented homosexual bathhouses in New Jersey. He initially told me he was a straight arrow. I got inoculated with his blood through a needle stick."

There was silence. Then Dr. Alford said, "Have you been tested for AIDS, Matt?"

"Yes, and I'm negative."

There was a sigh of relief around the table. Bill Burns muttered, "Man, what an ass-tightener. You can test the patient, and the doctors, but someone will creep through the woodwork. It's a public health problem, though, since there are millions in the United States who are already infected. What a ball-buster. I'm glad I'm quitting."

"I think you have to protect those who don't have the disease," said Matt. "In the past, if you got smallpox or tuberculosis, you were quarantined. Today, we're hiding the AIDS patients from public view, protecting privacy at the expense of public health."

"I agree. We have to stop the spread of the disease or we'll all be wiped out," said Andrews. "It could be a worldwide disaster."

"It is already," said Milstein. "You'll never totally wipe it out, because the disease is transmitted among adults in this country almost exclusively by two routes; sexual intercourse, and the sharing of contaminated needles by drug abusers."

"You'll never be able to prevent homosexuality," said Burns.

"Sex is here to stay," said Alford. "It's at the root of a lot of our problems. Read the newspapers. We have so many divorces in this country. Let's face it, the family structure is breaking up."

"Well, psychiatrists have not helped keep it together," said Andrews. "Most psychiatrists are all screwed up."

"No comment," said Alford. "On second thought, thanks a lot."

"I think all AIDS patients and all doctors who have AIDS should be identified," said Milstein. "Nobody in their right mind is going to go into any branch of surgery in the future. Hell, the other day I saw one of the bone surgeons doing a hip replacement. The air in the room had to be sterilized and cleansed—at tremendous cost I might add—and the surgeon had to wear a space suit that probably cost as much as the one they used to go to the moon.

"As they drilled the hip and bone joint, blood was spewing all over the place. Since you can't identify the patient with AIDS unless they give you permission to do a blood test, all the surgeon would need is a little break in the system, and if the patient had AIDS and the surgeon took one deep breath, he'd have the virus in his lungs. He also has to wear special rubber gloves, which can break very easily. All he would need is a break in the skin or a little eczema and he'd be inoculating himself with the AIDS virus."

"If you identify all the AIDS patients and doctors with AIDS, they'd all be discriminated against," said Alford.

"That's a bunch of crap," said Burns. "Who's really being discriminated against? Those who have the disease or those who don't? The patients I feel sorry for are those who got bad blood transfusions or transplanted organs with AIDS, or the children of mothers who have AIDS. These are the innocent bystanders. On balance, the rest of the AIDS patients knew what they were doing. They chose their own lifestyles and they created their own problems."

"They still get deathly sick just like anyone else," said Snow, "and if you're a dedicated physician you have to take care of them."

"There's an administrator telling the doctors what to do again," said Bill Burns.

"That's right," said Andrews. "But there's nothing in the Hippocratic Oath that says I have to take care of patients who put me and my family at excessive risk. If I die from AIDS that I contracted from a patient who I can't identify or who lies to me, who's going to take care of my family? If they identify themselves so I can protect myself adequately, I'll be glad to take care of them."

"Why don't you guys change the subject," said Steve Walters. "It's too goddamned depressing! Besides, and this may be a first, we all agree! Test the doctors, test the patients who are being admitted to the hospital, so the hospital personnel can protect themselves. That's only fair!

"If you want something else to talk about, why don't you guys figure out ways of keeping the cost of medical care down. Doctors are being blamed for that problem, too. The cost of health care is going out of sight and AIDS certainly isn't reducing it. The cost of getting rid of medical waste and contaminated instruments and clothing has gone sky high.

"Because of the AIDS problem and hepatitis, the government and patients have mandated stringent controls to protect medical personnel from blood-borne waste products and utensils: needles, surgical instruments and clothing that may have become contaminated. The price tag for that one is eight-hundred million dollars, thanks to OSHA."

"Well, you have to protect the people in the workplace," said Snow, "and the patients you work on."

"I couldn't agree more, but unless we cut the cost of health care immediately, we're going to break the bank. There won't be money left for anything else," said Steve Walters.

"That's right," said Matt, "but in the process of doing just that, we're creating more paperwork, more new equipment costs, more jobs for administrators and inspectors. The biggest new cost is paying for disposal of waste and finding a safe place to get rid of it. We're creating a whole new business."

"Let's face it, you doctors are one of the big reasons health care costs are going out of sight," said Snow. "Don't blame it all on big business. Neurosurgeons get six-thousand dollars for one five-hour case. Heart surgeons get eight-thousand dollars for heart surgery they can do in four or five hours. Coronary bypass surgery is the most common operation done today in this hospital. The price for doing that surgery should be reduced—instead it's going up! Hand surgeons get fifteen-hundred dollars for carpal tunnel operations on the wrist that take them thirty minutes to do. One of our hand surgeons does ten to twenty of these a day. Anesthesiologists charge ten to fifteen dollars a minute—portal to portal—for their services, eye doctors zap the eyes with a laser and charge two-thousand dollars and the list goes on and on. So I don't think I'll listen to a lot of bullshit about big business being the only bad guy."

"Wait a minute," said Andrews. "Doctor's fees only play a small part of health care costs—about twenty-five percent of the total cost. Big business has been taking over medicine for the past twenty-five years. When I started practice there were two administrators in this hospital and both were doctors. The size of the hospital hasn't changed and yet now, there are fourteen vice presidents and probably thirty assistant vice presidents, each getting a good salary. Administrators proliferate like flies. And let's not leave out the insurance companies. The HMOs and PPOs and IPOs were all supposed to reduce the cost of medical care. All they did was make more new jobs. The insurance industry wouldn't be in the health care business if they didn't make money, just look at how much it costs them to advertise—so naturally their premiums are going out of sight. The insurance companies have no controls—they're not telling about their profits. Today a lot of young people have to decide whether they'll eat or pay their health insurance. That's why so many of them are going bare."

"There are some bright spots. What about managed health care or managed competition?" asked Snow.

"Managed health care is a big fake and grossly inefficient," said Bill Milstein.

"How so?"

"Whenever you have a clerk or a nurse on the other end of the phone, telling a doctor when he should admit a patient, how long the patient should stay in the hospital, and what tests he can order, there's something wrong with the system. Managed health care means that the insurance company selects a group of doctors to work for them to eliminate competition."

"There's another reason for high health care costs. The insurance companies are just like the hospitals. They've got five times as many administrators as they need," said Milstein. "They need a General Motors cleanout. There's too much middle management."

"What about people who can't afford health insurance?" asked Burns. "Let's face it. We're not covering the populace adequately. We're not taking care of the poor. We're the only modern country that doesn't have National Health Care. The rich are the only ones getting excellent care. *There are thirty-six million Americans who have no health insurance.* Many of the uninsured are young people who can't get jobs or who only work part-time."

"Here! here!" the group answered in unison.

"So who's going to pay for health insurance?" asked Snow.

"Everyone is going to have to chip in," said Burns. "The insurance companies shouldn't be allowed to cherry-pick who they'll cover. And ultimately, the rates for health insurance should all be the same. They should not be based on health status, age, sex, occupation, or geographic location."

"Bill, who's going to set those rates?" asked Walters, "It can't be the insurance companies. They'll set them high enough to continue making their big profits."

"A cross-section representative group of the people should set those rates, limiting profit margins," said Andrews. "The government may have to pass laws to regulate the insurance industry. The ideal would be to have one payer and one collector of the premiums. If the federal government didn't want to handle it, the states could do it. However, the rules and methods would have to be set by federal laws so there would be no hanky-panky."

"How are you going to make them more efficient?" asked Alford.

"Stop the paperchase," replied Andrews. "Come over to my office and see how much time is spent filling out forms. There are over fifteen-hundred insurance companies in the health care business. Most of them require a specific form for their claims. There should be one simplified claim form for all the insurance companies."

"Amen to that, brother," they all replied in unison.

"I'd throw the bums out. There should be a clean sweep of the people who run the health care business," said Bill Burns.

"Burns, you're a nihilist, you know that?" said Snow.

Bill Burns smiled and pressed on. "They've got the biggest lobby in Washington. The lawyers, insurance companies, drug companies, and health care suppliers would scream bloody murder. We could never pass a law for National Health Care. There are too many vested interests that would be destroyed. The politicians wouldn't have the guts to pass it."

"Why haven't the HMOs and PPOs and IPOs helped in reducing costs?" asked Alford.

"Because they're more like insurance companies than not. Some have been bought up by the insurance companies," said Andrews. "They're wolves in sheep's clothing. They were supposed to reduce the cost of health care. All they did is create more jobs. Health care is a profitable business. The cost of medical care could be reduced immensely if that big profit was taken away."

"Aren't you guys exaggerating the role of the insurance industry?" asked Snow. "After all, they seem to pay all our bills and yours too, for that matter. I will admit they're slow in paying the hospital."

"They pay the hospital because half of the corporaters of the hospitals are either lawyers or are from the insurance industry," said Steve Walters. "It's like the fox watching the chicken coop."

"That's hitting below the belt," said Snow. "There are people of good character in this business. Sure, we've had a lawyer and some successful businessmen as heads of our hospital board. Would you want us to have a truck driver running the board?"

"Worth a shot. Might shake things up," said Steve Walters.

"You sound kind of bitter, Steve."

"I haven't even started. My bitch isn't just with the insurance industry for the high cost of health care. I have a bone to pick with those new companies in biomedical research that are going out of sight on the stock exchange. My patients can't afford to pay for the expensive drugs they're producing. Let's face it, a lot of the basic biomedical research has been subsidized by the United States taxpayers. The public should have the right to buy their products for a reasonable price."

"Examples. Let's hear some," said Burns.

"Taxpayers have given billions to the National Institutes of Health to discover and test new drugs. Once they are developed private drug companies get licensed to produce and market the drugs at a high price tag for the consumer—for example; AZT, DDC and DDI, used in AIDS treatment.

"I can give you a list the length of your arm," said Steve. "One monthly injection of Carboplatinum, an anticancer drug, can cost one-thousand dollars. Some people have diseases that require frequent blood transfusions. There's a new drug that can treat anemia, but it's too expensive and the patients can't afford it. One bottle of hyperalimentation costs thirty-five dollars—intravenous nutrition for patients who have lost weight. Tamoxifen, the anticancer drug used for breast disease, continues to increase in cost. No one can afford Taxol, the new drug for ovarian cancer. The cost is out of sight. The poor can't afford these drugs. Some of the drug houses are scalping the public. The drug companies can charge whatever the traffic will bear."

"I agree with Steve," said Matt. "I recently did a pancreatectomy on a Medicare patient and was told to discharge him before he was ready to go home. That's managed care for you. Sometimes, following a pancreatectomy, a fistula develops and drains to the outside skin. I had a patient who had one of those fistulas. I was told by Medicare to discharge him. I started the patient on Somatostatin to dry up the fistula. The next day, I got a phone call from the patient. 'Hey, Doc, you're a terrific surgeon, but I can't afford the prescriptions you write.'

"What do you mean? I asked. The guy says he went to the drugstore to pick up the medicine and they wanted nine-hundred and fifty dollars for thirty vials of Somatostatin. I called the druggist and he said, 'I don't tell you what to charge for your surgery. You're not going to tell me what to charge for my drugs. That's the going price.' "

"That's the marketplace," said Hammon. "How much did the visiting nurse association charge for administering the injections?"

"One hundred and ten dollars a day for a five-minute visit."

"Oh, brother," said Walters. "That's almost four thousand dollars for thirty days, just for giving a shot."

"We haven't even gotten to the medical-surgical supply business," said Burns.

"Let's get to it, then," said Snow.

"At the hospital we used to sterilize all our equipment in a central area. Today, everything is prepackaged and disposable. It costs an arm and a leg to dress a nurse or surgeon prior to entering the operating room.

"Intraoperative equipment costs have also gone out of sight. Don't get me wrong. The medical advancements are great—special stapling devices for sewing the bowel or blood vessels together. Metal clips to close the skin, instead of sutures, expedite closure, but they're disposable and expensive. When I started practice, one suture with a needle on it cost thirty-two cents. Today it costs ten times as much."

"There's less chance of infection with disposable equipment," said Snow. "There's been progress using the new operative devices."

"I'll agree with that," said Burns. "Johnson & Johnson, U.S. Surgical, and other companies have developed some fancy devices that allow the surgeon to take out the gallbladder without a big incision. Some instruments help in doing hysterectomies and sewing the bowel together with staplers."

"You haven't mentioned anything about malpractice insurance increasing the cost of medical care," said Andrews.

"Here we go," said Burns. "That's a big bag of worms!"

"I've avoided that," said Matt. "But I should say something about it. After all, I was tarred and feathered by the media before my malpractice case went to trial. And when it looked as if the opposition was going to lose the case, I had to sign a paper stating I wouldn't sue them because they had instituted a frivolous case.

"When I started practice, I paid nothing for malpractice insurance. Today, it's one-third of my salary. In some states, like Florida, it's over one-hundred thousand dollars for coverage. When lawyers say paying for malpractice doesn't increase health care costs, they're crazy! And they know it! Any costs that are added to practicing medicine are transferred to the patient's tab. The patients who sue aren't the only ones who benefit from malpractice awards. The lawyers get between thirty to forty-five percent of the settlement. The insurance companies also make money from insuring the doctors. They also charge big bucks for defending the doctors.

"I once had a prominent malpractice lawyer say to me, 'All I want is one big malpractice settlement. A figure around ten million would be fine, and then I'll retire on the 3.5.' "

"Malpractice insurance was developed to benefit the patient," said Milstein. It looks as if all it benefits are the lawyers. We're the only country in the world that has such high malpractice benefits. Most doctors will agree that accidents do occur, but there should be a limit on awards for pain and suffering. There are just too many frivolous lawsuits out there.

"It's been estimated the threat of malpractice lawsuits adds fifty-six million dollars a year in insurance premiums to the nation's health care bill and another fifteen billion dollars in the cost of defensive medical studies that doctors have to use to protect themselves. Those billions could be better spent to reduce the premiums of health care costs. Just mention national health care to malpractice lawyers and they go pale."

"How would you change malpractice costs?" asked Snow.

"I'd go into a no-fault system with an arbitration board. If an accident happens the patient gets paid—not the lawyer. Pain and suffering would have a cap. Instead of having malpractice insurance paid for by the doctors, have an airline insurance system—when you fly, you pay. When every patient is admitted to the hospital, they pay. A sum of money is put into a trust system in case an accident occurs."

"You guys have been doing all the talking and pointing the finger. I'd like a rebuttal," said Snow.

"You've got the floor," said Alford.

"I've told you before, the way to keep costs down is to form a Mayo Clinic-type of organization in this hospital. Let the hospital handle your paperwork."

"That's ridiculous," said Andrews. "The hospital can't handle its own paperwork. Their billing system stinks. It takes them six months, or longer, to send a bill and even then it's a miracle if it's correct. There's always a lot of padding in the bill—charging big amounts for services not rendered—so-called "miscellaneous charges." I found out my patients were being charged extra so the hospital's surgical heart program could get off the ground. They never informed the patients. They just tacked it onto their bills."

"Well, we have one of the best heart programs in the country now," said Snow.

"Oh, so the end justifies the means," said Matt. "I did a bladder resection on a patient and created an ileal bowel reservoir to collect the urine. The hospital charged the patient nine-hundred and fifty dollars for a Dacron ileal vessel graft that's used in vascular surgery. I didn't even use that graft. It took three months to correct that mistake in the hospital billing office."

"The reason the hospital wants to form a Mayo Clinic is so the hospital can keep the income generated by the doctors," said Andrews.

"Mr. Snow, you still haven't told us why the white linen on the breakfast table," said Alford.

Snow looked at the group, obviously concentrating on picking his words carefully. He had been deflated by the doctors sitting around the table more than once.

"Well, Dr. Bill Burns, our former chief of urology, is retiring to Arizona and has served this hospital well, though it pains me somewhat to admit it.

"Dr. Kendall, our senior cancer surgeon, who has done surgery at this hospital for over thirty years, told me he is quitting surgery also.

"I thought it would be appropriate to have white linen for this last breakfast of the Inner Sanctum Brain Trust. Before we break up, I think we ought to ask Dr. Burns and Dr. Kendall to briefly summarize their thoughts about the future. Why don't you go first, Bill."

"OK, but you're not going to like what I have to say."

"Oh, my," said Snow. "It won't be the first time."

"I'm afraid we're moving toward complacency and mediocrity in medicine. The doctors have lost control of how they practice medicine. The insurance industry has been overhauling the nation's health care system without any progress for years, trying to force the doctors into a prepaid, closed panel, group practice. They call it managed health care or managed competition and they pick the doctors for the system as they pocket their profits. There are too many insurance companies out there not taking care of the poor. Small business cannot pay for the cost of insuring their employees, and giving tax credits to pay for health insurance is no good if you don't have a job or if you only have a part-time job.

"In this country, it's everyone's right to have equal access to health insurance and equal care. What the health insurance companies have done is to make an organizational entrapment of our health care delivery system. Doctors have no quarrel with so-called group practice and its right to exist. They do have a quarrel when it exists to the exclusion of other systems, and when public funds are used to promote one system over the other. It has come to that. Maybe the government should be running the show. I'll sit down now, and thank you gentlemen for your attention."

"That certainly was a mouthful," said Snow. "I'm glad you're retiring."

"Would you like to make a few comments, Matt?" asked Snow.

Matt stood up and looked around the table. The men sitting at the table had been friends and adversaries for the past 30 years. He glanced over at Mr. Snow.

"Before I comment about what I think is on the horizon for medicine, I think we owe a debt of gratitude to Mr. Snow, our C.E.O., and to all the doctors in the past who have helped make Whitestone Hospital one of the finest hospitals in the country. It took a lot of sweat and intestinal fortitude to accomplish what has happened here at this institution. Medicine has had more advances in the past thirty years than in the whole past century."

"Here! Here!" the group responded in unison.

"I'll start my comments by saying if it ain't broke, don't fix it. Having said that, I think it's high time we take a cold, unimpassioned look at this enforced medical care system that is being thrust upon us. Is prepaid, closed-panel, group practice the best and most economical system to meet all the health needs of a diversified America? Who should run it?

"The insurance industry has had ample time to lead us and has failed. Should the government run the system? Are we, as patients, willing to lose the freedom of choosing our own physician? Should the fee-for-service principle be abolished, and all physicians salaried? How do we control the cost of new drugs and sophisticated equipment? Should we eliminate malpractice costs and have a no-fault system of payment for injury? How do we cut administrative costs and the so-called paper chase? How do we eliminate the skyrocketing costs and salaries of the leaders? Why is there a differential medicare payment to doctors? Why are some doctors allowed to charge more? Why should there be a geographical difference in payment? Shouldn't it be one national fee scale or no fee scale at all? If we salary all physicians, how are we going to determine what that salary should be? How do we get rid of some of our professional medical politicians who have gotten us into this mess? The medical establishment—our so-called leaders—should we throw them all out? There's gridlock in medicine, also. We have too many people who have never practiced medicine, trying to tell the doctors what to do."

Mr. Snow broke into Matt's talk.

"Are we going to be allowed to ask you two veteran doctors questions?"

"Why not? We won't be practicing anymore, so we won't have to worry about reprisal," said Matt with a smile.

"Well, if you're so smart, how would you improve the system then?" asked Snow.

"Right off the bat I'd start at the top. I'd appoint a doctor as the head administrator of this hospital. You'd have a job, but you wouldn't be the boss."

"Why would you do that?"

"To improve communications between the doctors who are out there in the arena taking care of patients and the personnel working in the white ivory tower."

"What else would you do?" asked Milstein.

"I'd go right at the heart of the problem in Washington, DC. I'd separate the Health, Education, and Welfare Departments and have one single Health Department headed by a doctor who's been in the arena—in other words a *Secretary of Health*."

"What's wrong with the way it is now?

"We've got Ph.D.s with political science, Ph.D.s with economics degrees, and lawyers telling doctors what's wrong with the system. I don't see any doctors or lay personnel telling the legal departments (Attorney General's Office) in Washington what to do. They have their own little closed fraternity directing the traffic and making the laws. That's the main reason we have gridlock in Washington. How many lawyers wrote the Constitution of the United States? Not very many. The Constitution was drawn up by merchants, manufacturers, capitalists, and only a few lawyers.

"Unless doctors who have been out in private practice in the arena practicing medicine are allowed to play a role in setting policies for health care, the health care system will be destroyed and mediocrity will take its place.

"No one in their right mind is going to be willing to take the prolonged frustration and pay the price to become a good surgeon (15 years of training) because the enjoyment of practicing the difficult art of surgery will be destroyed. No one will want to take the stress of going into the surgical arena on a daily basis when the rewards are taken away.

"Medicine is like the Bill of Rights that followed the ratification of the Constitution. Managed competition and managed health care take away the patient's freedom of choice as to who takes care of them. The insurance industry's response to that is that they will let you have freedom of choice but at a reduced rate set by the insurance company—that discriminates against the poor who have to go with the cheapest method because they can't afford freedom of choice at a high price.

"These are just a few questions that have to be openly discussed and decided in the near future."

"It's too bad the newspaper's health reporters aren't around here to hear you two guys talk," said Andrews. "They might find out what the world is really like. Matt, what are your plans for the future?"

"Well, I've had two careers in my life, so far. First, I left college in my sophomore year to become a navy torpedo bomber pilot in the Atlantic and Pacific during World War II. Then, using the G.I. Bill of Rights, I went back to school and became a surgeon.

"It may sound corny, but I wanted to give something back. We fought that war to save this country. I wanted to practice surgery to improve it. And it's been a great experience, but our meeting here this morning has made it clear that we've lost track of our values, even our common sense of proportion and decency. I've never been afraid to say what I think."

"This much we know," said Burns. "So what are your plans?"

"I'm going to write," said Matt. "And make it my goal to tell people what modern medical practice is all about—also ways to improve it."

"Well," said Burns, "you've got all the material you need right in this room."

"You know," said Matt, "you're right."

Epilogue

A SURGEON'S THOUGHTS

I AM NOW A SENIOR attending surgeon at Whitestone Hospital, which gives me a certain amount of reverence and respect. I have been in the surgical arena for many years and have fought the fight, much like the gladiators of Roman times. Many of the fights were not easy. My fight was against the ravages of disease, usually cancer, using my surgical blade, attempting to cut out the cancer before it spread and destroyed the host.

Great strides in medicine and surgery have been made during my lifetime—new drugs (chemotherapy) have come on the horizon and radiation methods have been dramatically improved. Sophisticated diagnostic equipment is now being used, such as mammography, CT scans, magnetic resonance imaging machines, and ultrasound. Treatment methods have changed in surgery: heart-lung bypass machines enable surgeons to operate on the coronary vessels and valves; lithotriptors pulverize kidney stones; lasers cut and coagulate tissues more precisely; kidney dialysis machines prolong life after kidney destruction. Kidneys, hearts, lungs, and multi-organs are being transplanted—even islet cells of the pancreas so that diabetics will no longer be insulin dependent.

A new Star Wars surgery is developing. New techniques are challenging the old—such as laparoscopic procedures for gallbladders, hysterectomies, appendectomies, hernias, and lung resections.

Invasive radiologists are now working with cardiologists to do angioplasties on the blood vessels of the heart and challenging the heart surgeons. Lasers are now being used in treating prostates.

I have no regrets for having chosen surgery for my lifetime profession. I've learned as a surgeon that the human body is the same whether you are white, black, oriental, or a mixture of races. When I use my surgical blade to cut into the human body, the contents are always the same. The only difference is between male and female. Surgery helped me eliminate my own prejudices—it was an eye-opener for me—a great equalizer.

I have enjoyed the challenge and the stress associated with surgery. I know someday I will miss it. I once talked to an older surgeon who had retired. "Do you miss going into the surgical arena?"

"Of course I do!" he replied. "At first I missed it a great deal. I actually missed the nervousness and stress that I felt before I entered the operating room."

I thought about that—I still get nervous every time I go into the operating room. Perhaps, if a surgeon doesn't get nervous, he's chosen the wrong profession and might be the surgeon to avoid.

I often said a silent prayer before the start of a critical operation. "Dear God, please guide my brain and my hands so that I can help this patient get well."

The prayer didn't always work—if the patient died, I felt guilty—as if I might not have done my job right—that I had not prepared myself properly for the challenge. I would get depressed.

I thought about that prayer as I got older, and I decided that it was really a selfish prayer—if everything went well, I would be one of the beneficiaries and my practice would flourish.

I decided to change the prayer. "Dear God, may you bless this patient so that he or she may get well."

In my own mind, I feel I won the battle of the surgical arena many times—but there were also times when I lost. I know in my heart that those surgeons who follow in my footsteps will accept the challenge of the surgical arena and there will be new Star Wars on the horizon and new heights of accomplishment.